WE
CHOOSE
LOVE

PRAISE FOR *WE CHOOSE LOVE*

"*We Choose Love* invites the reader to deepen their level of intimacy with themselves by weaving spirituality, cutting-edge research, ancient wisdom, and deep listening. This is a nourishing love letter to the soul that inspires all who read it. Kristen D'Amato is a living example of the work."

MARLA MATTENSON, MA
CEO & Founder of the Ethical Sales Institute
Creator of the Ethical Sales Process

"Kristen D'Amato presents a framework of mind-body wellness to inspire greater awareness, emotional balance, and connection toward oneself and others while living with chronic conditions. *We Choose Love* offers insights into healing pathways by introducing philosophy, science, personal vignettes, simple assessment tools, and self-care practices. Readers are invited to reflect, assess, and explore different facets of their lifestyle in ways that are meaningful to them."

DEVORAH CURTIS, PHD
Department Chair, Mind-Body Medicine
Saybrook University

"As we continue to navigate the collective traumas of the triple pandemics, it is beneficial to ground oneself in love. The constantly changing conditions of our times and their intrinsic edge states invite the reader to explore balance, mind-body connection, and well-being through practices curated with love by author Kristen D'Amato."

DR. GINA BELTON
Mentor. Teacher. Ancestor. End of life Midwifery
Contemplative End of Life Care Specialization, Saybrook University
President, APA Division 32 Society for Humanistic Psychology

"*We Choose Love* speaks directly to the soul and has real potential to change people's lives. Within one month, I was eating completely plant-based, had come off medications I had been taking for years, and was no longer experiencing uncomfortable physical symptoms that had been impacting my daily life for a very long time. Emotionally, I felt clearer and freer than I ever remembered feeling. Changes began to occur that I had dreamed about but hadn't been able to envision actualizing. This book is a profoundly important body of work that offers an expansive understanding of what healing can look like. I would even say it has the potential to radically change the way humanity orients itself around health, healing, and well-being."

VANESSA OWEN, MDIV
Senior Research Services, Dept. of Family Medicine
University of Colorado School of Medicine
Hospice & Pediatric Trauma Chaplain, Children's Hospital Colorado

"Kristen D'Amato guides us on a heart-centered journey that incorporates ancient wisdom, practical and empowering strategies, and real-life, modern miracles of healing through adversity. A highly recommended reading for anyone unwilling to give up hope during challenging times."

DR. CARLOS SANTO, NMD
Core Faculty, Department of Mind-Body Medicine
Saybrook University

An empowering approach
to chronic conditions & beyond

WE
CHOOSE
LOVE

REDEFINING our RELATIONSHIP to HEALING

KRISTEN D'AMATO

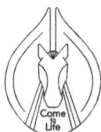

Come to Life
Los Angeles, CA

This book is not intended as a substitute for the medical recommendations of physicians, mental health professionals, or other health-care providers. Rather, it is intended to offer information to help the reader cooperate with physicians, mental health professionals, and health-care providers in a mutual quest for optimum well-being. We advice readers to carefully review and understand the ideas presented and to seek the advice of qualified professionals before attempting to use them.

All names and identifying details of the individuals in this book have been changed to protect their privacy.

Published 2023

Cover and book design by Linsey Dodaro

Printed in the United States of America

Library of Congress Cataloging-in-Publication Data
Names: D'Amato, Kristen, author.
Title: We choose love: redefining our relationship to healing / Kristen D'Amato.
Identifiers: LCCN 2023905995 (print) | ISBN 979-8-218-17705-8 (softcover)
Subjects: LCSH: Health. | Self-help.

10 9 8 7 6 5 4 3 2 1

CONTENTS

Dear Reader:

I hope this book will activate an expansion of love in your heart by reverberating the truth of what your soul knows to be true – we are multi-dimensional beings housed temporarily in a physical body that have come here to love and evolve. May this book be a guide, inviting you on a journey of reconnection and remembering. May *the Wheel of Whole Body Healing* awaken a resonance of hope and healing. May the stories illuminate great possibilities. May the exercises be an entryway, empowering you to listen to your inner wisdom and be guided by its light.

In Love & Service,

Kristen D'Amato

FOREWORD

At the time of the release of this book, it is estimated that over 60% of adults in the United States have a chronic illness, while over 40% have two or more, and 12% have five or more[1]. The number of U.S. adults with chronic illness is projected to reach 170 million by 2030[2]. Chronic illness accounts for 70 percent of all deaths in the U.S.[3], and chronic illness and mental illness care account for 90% of $4.1 trillion in U.S. health care spending[4]. Despite this alarmingly high incidence of illness and the enormous amount of money dedicated to understanding and treating it, patients often go years or decades without answers or relief.

As frightening as this picture is to imagine, it is even more frightening to experience. I am one of over 40% of people who have multiple chronic illnesses, and I am also someone who went decades undiagnosed, many of those years spent going from one doctor to another, dismissed as anxious and feeling completely unseen in my struggles. I'm also a researcher who is many years into my own research on the lived experiences of people with chronic conditions. It is not just my own experiences that haunt me. Every time I am faced with statistics like the ones above, I hear the voices of my participants, many dismissed and disempowered by medical professionals, most receiving inadequate care. They remain unseen as well.

I met Kristen in 2016; she was an instant friend to me, the kind that you meet and are sure you were supposed to know. But it is not my immediate connection with her that I want to share about here. It is that she has given me something that many providers, both Western and alternative, could not. She has listened. She has seen me for who I am. She has been willing to ask me what I know and understand and what healing means to me. With so many with chronic conditions going unseen by doctors and other healthcare professionals and rates of chronic illnesses increasing, I think the new paradigm of healing and patient care must be one of listening, believing, and joining patients on their searches for wellness.

This book is written to join patients on their journeys of healing. In my research, I discovered two main states of awareness between which those with chronic conditions oscillate: identified awareness and integrated awareness. When one is in identified awareness, they are consumed by their symptoms. Their world feels small and dark, and it is hard to think about anything else. For conditions in which symptoms flare, it is almost impossible to avoid shifting into this state during a flare. Indeed, sometimes the body is so loud, it is hard to hear anything else. Integrated awareness is a broader awareness; it is how we feel when we remember that we are whole people with interests, desires, and gifts. When we are in integrated awareness, we may still be sick, but we are people in which sickness is just a part of our experience, along with so many other things. Integrated awareness is a state of wellness, and I absolutely believe one can be both ill and well. Many of us with chronic conditions spend years, even lifetimes, trying to find our way into a more integrated awareness more of the time. I have been ill since I was a child, and it has taken me decades to discover the things that help me move into that state and that help me return to it when I am suffering. What I believe Kristen offers in this book is a roadmap of some of the ways one might shift into this broader awareness and experience more joy, pleasure, healing, and wellness, whether in place of illness as part of a radical healing process or in conjunction with illness, as a set of tools one can lean on again and again as they learn to live a fuller life just as they are. If you are someone with a chronic condition, diagnosed or not, or you love someone with illness, I hope you find inspired and empowering ideas to support you on the pages that follow.

Emily Cashwell, PhD

INTRODUCTION

Happiness is the great work,
though every heart must first become a student
To one who really knows
about Love.

HAFIZ

14th century Sufi poet

T his is a story of love. It is not the typical love story where "person meets person," they fall deeply in love at first sight, and after many trials and tribulations live happily ever after. Though it is not that different either.

This is a story of the most profound love of all. It *is* a story of love at first sight. Yet as quickly as we recognize our true love, we forget the connection ever existed. We experience many years of challenges caused by forgetting our love. We have hints of memories that keep us yearning for a connection we know is possible, but don't remember how to find. Around every corner, new opportunities await that will slightly awaken the love we once felt. Glimmers of hope arise, but mostly there is a feeling that lies dormant in our cells, buzzing in the distance, calling us to remember. This is our human experience. It is the same for every one of us. We spend our lives searching for true love. Though our love has many names, the essence is the same for us all. It is a deep knowing that we are source energy. Every part of us is one with the creative spirit of all that exists. We are one. There is no separation. We are the love we are seeking!

WHY CHOOSE LOVE?

Imagine if every moment of every day on this beautiful planet, we spent believing without a moment of doubt that we were worth receiving every wish that our hearts desired. We had material items that filled us with pleasure, our health was consistently in an optimum state of vitality, our relationships were fulfilling beyond our wildest dreams, and our livelihood was deeply satisfying because we were sharing our gifts and adding value to the world. Sounds magnificent, doesn't it? What do you think is preventing us from living this life of opulence, joy, and satisfaction?

The only thing preventing us is the belief that we are unworthy of this degree of love, support, and happiness. This is the biggest fallacy and the most sabotaging belief that human beings have. To embody the wholeness of who we truly are, we must embrace our worthiness and be gentle with ourselves. The question then becomes, how do we acknowledge and integrate the deepest, shadowy parts of ourselves? The path is clear; it is through consistent acts of love.

In this book, I will be sharing a model of self-care I created called the *Wheel of Whole Body Healing*. It is alive and evolving. Its sole intent is to reduce suffering by creating freedom derived from self-awareness on the deepest levels possible. It is a working model that when used time and time again supports us to uncover and discover the truths and fears we have. Using this model as a guide helps us experience love in more profound ways than we ever have before. It is a model that expands with us, and for us.

The most significant contribution we can make during our time here on Earth is to love as fully as possible. Although this sounds simple, it requires continual commitment to integrity in our choices. As acceptance of ourselves expands, the more we are able to radiate magnificence through our unique expressions and share our splendid gifts with the world. How big are you willing to love? How big are you willing to love yourself? The answer is the same. We can only give love to another as much as we are willing to give love to ourselves. We can only receive love from another as much as we are willing to receive love from ourselves. Are you ready to be bold and brave? It requires courage to meet the tenderest parts of ourselves with care.

When we choose love, I mean really go for it, we live in a world where our dreams become our reality, where joy is as commonplace as the air we breathe, and love, oh love, comes to us endlessly from all directions with no bounds. When we choose love, we feel increasingly better in our bodies. Diseases can heal and illness can have less of an effect on us. When we choose love, we feel a deep connection with all life forms, and it becomes impossible for loneliness to linger. When we choose love, we walk alongside our beloveds with great reverence rather than collapse into co-dependency.

Though choosing love is simple, it is also a radical departure from the way most of us have lived our lives. It is certainly the opposite end of the spectrum from how many of us are taught to live. It takes passionate commitment, consistent action, and a receptivity to look at our blind spots. This requires meeting the unconscious roles within that blame, caretake, shame, and fear. As we welcome the parts of us we have feared back to our family table, healing occurs accompanied by new awareness and clarity. This enables monumental swells of love to pour graciously in.

The *Wheel of Whole Body Healing* is a guiding template for embarking on this journey of self-inquiry and discovery. It is a tool to inspire and awaken more connection with ourselves as we use it to reflect upon challenges and imbalances we are experiencing in our lives. The exercises are designed to awaken deeper listening and experiential awareness. Are you curious and open to learning from your body? Do you desire increasing your capacity to give and receive more love? Experiment with the exercises and see where they guide you. When the *Wheel* is put into practice, our world rapidly shifts as we recognize more clearly the divine orchestration we are a part of.

EVOLVING OUR PERCEPTION OF HEALING

These days our systems are heavily burdened by external environmental factors and internal debilitating patterns. Pollution of all types (chemical, emotional, spiritual, mental, pathogenic, etc.) has strained our bodies' healing capacities. Chronic illness is at a catastrophic high leaving many people feeling disempowered and suffering. We cannot control all harmful exposure, however, there is much we can do to limit exposure and build resilience.

New approaches are required for the depth of healing upon us. Conventional methods are not designed to address the complexities of many chronic conditions. This is evidenced by the statistics currently circulating in the medical research community. Additionally, the conventional medicine model is built on a mechanistic perspective, designed to fix that which is broken. It excels in the arena of infectious disease and physical traumas requiring repair. Chronic conditions are another beast altogether. They are often comprised of various interactions between many systems in the body. A whole-body approach is necessary to begin to understand the cause and healing path. In this book, the definition of whole-body is expanded beyond the integration of the systems of the physical body. It includes energetics within and far beyond the physical boundary of the body. It takes into consideration the physical (conventional medicine), energetic (eastern medicine), and liminal (traditional medicine) realms. It encompasses the knowing that we are relational beings, and all life impacts one another

The *Wheel of Whole Body Healing* addresses multiple threads that are influential factors for wellness. It is an orientation that embraces the body and disease from a place of multi-dimensional wisdom, combined with practical strategies to support the body and mind to move toward homeostasis. There are great surprises that lie at the bottom of the treasure chest of our suffering. We simply must have the courage to embrace the opportunity presented and explore that which is surfacing to heal.

ONE

THE WHEEL OF WHOLE BODY HEALING

When you help, you see life as weak.
When you fix, you see life as broken.
When you serve, you see life as whole.

DR. RACHEL NAOMI REMEN
Kitchen Table Wisdom

What if we viewed our pain and suffering as a gift? What if rather than be a victim to our bodies, we valued them as great storytellers with wisdom to be heeded that would lead us down the path of evolution toward a joyful life?

We are taught in American culture that we are victims of the world around us, and that life circumstances are something happening to us. While there is some truth to this, it is not the whole picture. This perspective has created a culture of deeply disempowered individuals. We have forgotten that we are also grand creators in this story of life and that we have come here with a great purpose—to love, to serve, and to evolve. As we more fully embrace the duality of the human experience as laden with traumatic events combined with an ever-available access to creative potential for envisioning options, we see that pain is inevitable, however suffering is not.

People have existed for centuries disconnected from the truth of who we are. Many of us have forgotten we are wildly creative, powerful souls temporarily housed in physical bodies. We have created systems built on the mistruth that what we see before us, our physical reality, is the only reality that exists or is relevant. Therefore, the support systems we have created are deeply flawed and fail to support us to fully thrive.

Our understanding of the human body mirrors this misunderstanding by encompassing only a narrow slice of who we are. There are so many aspects that are not addressed when looking at ailments and pains we are suffering from. How can healing happen if those that are giving and receiving care only address a few pieces of the thousand-piece puzzle we are?

The *Wheel of Whole Body Healing* is an ever-evolving system that *begins* to address the complexity of who we are. It is a model embedded with the inherent trust in the body's wisdom to be a great teacher. It is a model that encourages deep listening to this wisdom as a roadmap for our healing. It is a model that empowers rather than negates what we are feeling, where our intuition is honored, welcomed, and cultivated. In this model, we are the directors of our healing journeys, not disempowered recipients of temporary bandages.

We are individuals that are on our unique healing journeys during this lifetime. At the same time, we are all connected, participating in a grand evolution and healing of humanity. Each of us has a responsibility to show up the best way we know how to evolve ourselves, our lineages, and the collective in our time here on Earth. The *Wheel of Whole Body Healing* supports this pathway while providing greater insight into why pains and imbalances may be occurring. I believe it is possible to heal anything. This may be uncomfortable to hear. Some of us have experienced unbearable suffering. By saying this, it does not discount everything that has been tried before leading you to this moment. Healing is about the journey of becoming more in alignment and connection with our essence and our sense of place in the human collective. We are all on a path of remembering how to do this. Shifting our perspective on what it means to heal leads us on a trajectory exploring how extraordinary we are and reveals more of what is possible.

MENTAL WELLNESS

Why do we focus on mental illness rather than on mental wellness? This stigmatizes people as something being "wrong" with them. Have you ever wondered who is deciding what constitutes "normal" that whole systems are built upon? I frequently saw clients suffering from chronic anxiety. Many had been on medication and in the psychiatric system for years. They were repeatedly told there was *something wrong with them* and they were going to have to learn how to deal with it for the rest of their lives. The best-case proposal was constituted of strategies for coping with the problem.

Many years ago, I worked in a residential program as a teacher and house guardian for children transitioning from the psychiatric ward back into "normal" life. The program was a stepping-stone designed to give kids the skills and support to reintegrate back into their homes and lives. At the time, I was one of the few adults participating in meetings that did not have traditional psychiatric training that determined how to best support the kids. Most of them had come from households that were emotionally, physically, and/or sexually abusive. They had a variety of behavioral challenges that made it difficult for them socially. Some were self-abusive and hospitalized to protect them from hurting themselves. All the children were consistently taking an average of nine different psychiatric medications. There was a no-touch policy between those of us who worked there and the children, the exception being when we had to restrain one of them, so they didn't hurt themselves or another. In these meetings, the approach to supporting the kids was exclusively clinical. There was talk of adjusting medications, putting them on different task protocols, and different ways to train them via consequences. After some time, I began to chime in about two main things. The first is, why is all the attention focused on the children being the problem, rather than on the rehabilitation of the adults raising them? They experienced and witnessed so much abuse and yet they were accused of something being wrong with them. The second was, how can healthy reintegration be expected when they came in having experienced physical touch as traumatic and they are leaving here without us modeling loving touch for them. What kind of adult are they likely to become having either touch that hurts them or touch that restrains them as the basis for what is normal?

I initiated teaching yoga classes as part of the program to provide a safe container for positive touch. I also would give them a loving touch on the shoulder or a similar gesture when they accomplished a goal. This challenged many of the adults in the community. Fortunately, I had one supervisor who supported my methods, and he was able to talk with the others to see what transpired. Within a short period, I gained the trust of most of the children, and I became their go-to when they were in crisis. This inspired some changes in the parameters around adult-to-child interactions at this institution. Something as simple as treating them as human, instead of clinical diagnoses, as well as expressing love and appreciation, saved a life on multiple occasions.

I invite you to approach mental illness from a different perspective. One common pattern I saw in clients who presented with "mental illness" is that they were highly sensitive individuals. They came into this world with great perceptive abilities awakened and their families and communities did not understand the value of these gifts and how to nurture them. Unfortunately for the sensitive ones, they were quickly labeled and diagnosed as being other and categorized as having something "wrong" with them. They were often compartmentalized because there was not a greater understanding of how to best support them. A deep aspect of their suffering came from being excluded and feeling a foundational sense of not being good enough to receive love.

One of the first things I offered to clients suffering from mental health challenges was to explore shifting their perspective, often for the first time, to seeing their "illness" as a reflection of their gifts. Many times, this gift is heightened awareness and psychic abilities. This invitation alone often brought about profound healing. To consider themselves, even for a moment, as whole and not broken was deeply empowering.

This is not to dismiss that chemical imbalances occur that cause us to feel anxiety, depression, etc. Many factors contribute to symptoms of mental imbalance. It takes addressing *all* factors simultaneously to support transformation. This takes time and commitment on our part. Looking for someone to "fix" us with a diagnosis and medication may help some, or even all, the symptoms to subside. However, it is likely the root cause of the imbalance still exists. If so, it will express in another form. We need to get curious about what it is within us that contributes to our imbalances. This is true with physical symptoms as well.

PHYSICAL WHOLENESS

Many physical symptoms are manifestations of imbalances that began in the energy body. After a time of being left unattended, from a lack of awareness, the alarm has become louder and clearer. When I say physical symptoms, I do not mean trauma caused to the body such as a broken bone or a gunshot wound. I am referring to a wide variety of acute and chronic experiences that are the result of deep subconscious patterning, trapped emotional energy, ancestral lineage pain, and disempowerment.

Our bodies are master communicators. We need to remember how to understand the language they are speaking. If we can sense the voice of imbalance when it exists only in the subtler, energetic realms, perhaps we can prevent it from manifesting into physical form. At any rate, the sooner we listen to the symptoms in our physical bodies and honor the request to pay attention, the better our chance to minimize suffering.

THE WHEEL OF WHOLE BODY HEALING

The *Wheel of Whole Body Healing* is comprised of seven facets. Together, these facets begin to address the depth of what is affecting all aspects of our human experience, such as our physical and emotional states, our creativity, our relationships, and our work in the world.

In the following chapters, I discuss each of the seven facets and how they contribute to the roots of imbalance. I also share experiential stories to demonstrate both the significance of addressing a particular facet and how working with it manifested in real life. There are exercises woven throughout the book to support the implementation of these concepts and begin strengthening muscles of awareness. Lastly, at the end of the book, there is a list of resources and modalities that support each facet of the *Wheel*. We will find the greatest success in being conscious advocates for ourselves and wisely choosing specialists that support the different aspects with their expertise.

The seven facets of the *Wheel of Whole Body Healing*:

1. Unexpressed Emotional Energy
2. Feeding Our Light Body – Our Dietary Choices
3. Physical Ailments & Imbalances
4. Our Energy Fields
5. Healing Our Ancestral Lineage
6. Embodying Our Sexual Power
7. Empowerment Tools & Strategies

FULFILLING OUR LIFE'S PURPOSE

We have all come to this planet to fulfill our life's purpose and evolve. The details of how this happens are different for everyone. Each of us has a unique contribution that our soul brings. Our lives are the arena for remembering our essence and embodying it.

We often focus on the details of *what* to do for a job, rather than highlighting the gifts we bring forth as a soul. Once this is recognized, the details of how one chooses to manifest it on the physical plane (as a job) could look a million different ways. This depends on our inspirations from moment to moment. The core resonance remains true and steady regardless of the label put on the actions we perform. For example, at my core, I am a healer and a teacher. During my life thus far, whatever form my job has taken, I have effortlessly brought forth my gifts as a healer and teacher. The more I honor the truth of who I am, the more brilliantly my gifts shine through. This allows me to have a greater impact on the world. Sharing our unique brilliance is an empowering and meaningful aspiration for our lifetimes.

Our aches and pains can be representations that we are misaligned with our core values. They may be warning signals that we are ready to evolve. When we can take these opportunities and look at them head-on, as scary as they may be, we can make pivotal discoveries about our desires. This is a path to living in joy. A joyful life does not mean there are never any bumps, pains, or fear. On the contrary, it means we have the awareness that our suffering is a sign compelling us toward a deeper truth and aligning us more fully with our life's purpose. The *Wheel of Whole Body Healing* is a template for addressing suffering, heartbreaks, and imbalances. It is an orientation that becomes a lifestyle, for redefining our relationship to healing. I invite you to explore re-membering the truth of who you are and fall madly in love with the exquisite nature of your essence. Shall we begin?

EXERCISE

Listening Within - Sensing Subtle Energy

This is an introductory exercise to begin awakening your listening skills. The process will both ground you and cultivate awareness about what is happening inside your body at any given time. It is important to be *willing to listen* to what your body is communi-cating to hear the invitation to heal.

1. Find a comfortable seated position directly on the Earth, ideally with your shoes off.

2. Close your eyes and turn your attention inward.

3. Gently lengthen your breaths, inhaling and exhaling through your nose.

4. Allow your exhalations to be double the length of your inhalations. It doesn't need to be exact.

5. Spend 5-10 breaths settling into your breathing, so that it becomes effortless. If you can, allow yourself to relax.

6. Now turn your attention to the Earth beneath you. Feel the energy of Mother Earth connecting with your energy field. Know that you are held and safe. Allow this awareness to be an opening to connect with yourself and your body.

7. Notice any sensations in your physical body. Start with the obvious sensations and then tune in, even deeper, to the subtler sensations.

8. Do not try to understand or change anything. Simply observe what you are sensing. Do you notice areas of discomfort, tension, tingling, warmth, numbness, etc? Try to sense other sensations beyond the loudest ones.

9. Continue this exploration for as long as you want, knowing that each minute that passes allows a deeper, more grounded connection to what is happening inside of you.

TWO

UNEXPRESSED
EMOTIONAL ENERGY

The lens through which we perceive our reality is greatly colored by our emotional landscape and the patterning of our subconscious minds. Whether we fully express our emotions or not has a profound impact on the health of our physical bodies, our mental states, and our relationships. Expression does not mean spewing anger out at others, or even intellectually acknowledging we are upset. We must let emotional energy move through our bodies, and let the animal part of us shake it off. Dr. Peter Levine speaks beautifully to this in his body of work called *Somatic Experiencing*.[1]

Levine invited a fresh perspective on trauma healing in the seminal book, *Waking the Tiger*.[2] He said traumatic symptoms came from the "frozen residue of energy that has not been resolved or discharged; this residue remains trapped in the nervous system where it can wreak havoc on our bodies and spirits."[3] As human animals, we all experience varying degrees of trauma throughout our lifetime. As the chasm between humans and our animal nature has widened, our ability to move emotional energy through our nervous system has become debilitated or frozen. We have become dissociated from our instinctual responses by relying too heavily on our "human" intellectual responses. Intellectualizing emotional responses interrupts the physiological processes of our nervous system not allowing it to complete its cycle. As Levine stated, just because we distance ourselves from uncomfortable emotions, it does not mean they disappear. When we suppress our emotional responses, a vast array of symptoms can arise.

Practicing letting our instinctual selves complete the innate response to emotional and traumatic experiences has a significant impact on whether we succeed at letting joy and love lead our lives versus having the voice of doubt and fear become the dominant influencer of our choices. Unless we have consciously implemented strategies to make different choices, a subconscious, outmoded part of us can become the driver in our lives.

In addition to reactivating instinctual responses to emotions, becoming acquainted with the various parts of our internal landscape is crucial. Until we are aware of the existence and needs of the myriad of inner roles comprising our personality, we are subject to their often dominating reactions. Allying with our parts allows us to feel empowered in our lives and aligned with our values. It can be disheartening and confusing to be unaware of inner roles yet hear their voices so loudly. As we learn to love and accept the parts we have shamed and shunned, a relationship of tenderness and reciprocity is established. It also becomes easier to have levity and gentleness toward ourselves. The book, *No Bad Parts* by internal family systems pioneer Dr. Richard Schwartz, is an excellent reference to begin exploring and developing a skill set for welcoming our parts.[4]

Lucy's story is a clear example of how unexpressed emotional energy had a profound impact on the quality of her relationships. It also exemplifies how interrupted emotional responses translated into symptoms.

Lucy's Story – Selective Mutism

When I met Lucy, she was seven years old and had never spoken. She rarely used her voice for any type of vocal expression. She had been to many doctors and practitioners to find out why this might be happening. They did not find any physical evidence they felt would prevent her from being able to talk. Lucy was diagnosed with selective mutism, though they were still doing some testing to decide if she was autistic. She was also highly sensitive and psychic. It was clear upon meeting her that she was consciously connected with the unseen realms. She felt like she was half in her physical body and half in another plane of existence.

Lucy's parents were divorced. She lived with her father full-time. Her mother lived overseas, and they had barely seen one another since she left a few years prior. Her dad was a loving man, devoted to supporting his daughter. He hired me to do sessions with Lucy. At that time, I was practicing as an energy healer in the early stages of developing the *Wheel of Whole Body Healing*. The work I did with Lucy was heavily based on assisting the movement of a stockpile of emotional energy housed in her body and energy field. We addressed many layers of unexpressed emotions. In life, Lucy experienced overwhelm very quickly and consistently. During our first session, I could sense that she was likely trying to cope with her overwhelm by not talking. At the end of this first session, Lucy was beginning to speak words.

I continued working with Lucy for a total of five sessions. Every week she was talking more, as well as becoming more expressive with her body language. She already drew a lot of pictures, but the content of her artwork shifted. She was now "talking" through her artwork as well. She was drawing stories of how she was feeling. She was also giving hugs and offering physical affection significantly more than she had been. Her dad was astonished at the rapid change in Lucy's behavior. He was so grateful that she was expressing physical affection toward him and using language to ask for what she needed.

We came to an excellent pausing point about 6 weeks into our work together. Lucy was now ready to receive support from a speech therapist to exercise her vocal muscles and learn to enunciate clearly. She was progressively talking more and more each week. She had begun talking with her mother via video conferencing and her mom had arranged a trip to come to visit her. Though this was the beginning of a journey unfolding, Lucy and her family were experiencing more hope than they had in a long time.

Oftentimes, when we acknowledge and listen to the parts of ourselves that are grieving or afraid, the oppositional impact on our life subsides. When we ignore them because we are afraid or ashamed, they unconsciously gain control. When left unacknowledged, these parts of ourselves will sabotage our growth repeatedly. As we become more conscious of the parts we rejected and we discover what they need, they can become our allies. They originated from a need we had, often to protect ourselves from emotional pain. Although they had a role at the time they were created, that role has likely expired and needs to be redirected to continue benefiting us.

EXERCISE

Dialoguing with Your Inner Selves

Inner selves are the many parts of you that reside in your inner landscape. They take shape throughout your lifetime in response to different experiences. They have qualities and needs that often get unconsciously expressed. Learning how to recognize your inner selves, what they feel like, and what they need so you can welcome them as part of your team is required for mental wellness.

In this exercise, imagine you are holding someone or something you adore. It can be your child, a beloved pet, or anything you feel a tenderness toward. Connect with the sensation of this affection in your body. What does it feel like? Now, as you are meeting your inner selves, approach them with the same tenderness, openness, and patience you would this beloved being. This exercise can be done when guilt, shame, fear, or any other emotions arise that feel debilitating or prevent you from moving towards your goals.

1. Find a comfortable seat or position. Plant both feet firmly on the ground. Center yourself by taking steady, easeful breaths into your heart.

2. As you breathe into your heart space, notice the part of you that is unconditionally loving, kind, gentle, and nurturing. What does this inner self look like? Feel like? Stay present with this wise self as long as you want.

3. When you are ready, continue staying connected with your wise self and call forth the part of yourself you want to speak with. You can try making a request such as, "I'd like to speak with the part of myself that feels guilty about…" and then listen. Or, you can notice the part of your body that has a sensation when you have a strong emotional response to something that is aligned with your goals. Perhaps you can already sense the age of an inner self and you can call them forth this way.

4. Have the most conscious, empowered part of yourself ask a prompting question such as, "are you willing to share why you are upset?" or "what do you need from me right now?"

5. Listen for the first answer that comes. Do not think about this. It is not a logical exercise. Trust the process and get curious.

6. You may continue to ask questions *if* the self you are speaking with wants to share. It may require patience as you rebuild trust with the inner self that is emerging. This might look like sitting lovingly and curiously with this part on multiple occasions before they are ready to communicate.

7. Once you have gained clarity about their needs and you have allowed them to fully express (journaling can be an excellent way to let a part express,) you might want to ask what they need to be your ally in whatever topic you were sensing resistance around. You may need to give them another "job" if the one they have been doing is

no longer helping you. What is their skill set and what can they do instead that will help you move toward your desired goals?

8. Once you feel complete, reassure this inner self with loving, grateful words and gestures. Let them know they are safe, loved, and welcome.

This is a simple, yet powerful and illuminating exercise. By allowing our inner selves to be heard, we learn a lot about why we get triggered in certain situations and how to tend to our needs when this happens. As we practice this exercise, we begin to establish trust and cultivate a sense of safety that we provide for ourselves. It is in this practice that we shift away from looking to others to create safety for us and we are empowered to provide this need to ourselves.

PATTERNS OF COMMUNICATION

Unexpressed emotional energy stored in parts of the body is one cause of imbalance leading to symptoms. Another influence is the learned patterns of communication surrounding emotional responses. Once we have established which emotion (often associated with an inner self that has unmet needs) is causing discomfort, and we have awareness of the communication pattern that triggers this emotional response, we can become mindful about making different choices in the moment when we recognize an undesirable pattern being activated. Our bodies will often give us a reminder with a physical flare-up or familiar, uncomfortable sensation this is about to happen. Attuning our listening to our bodies so that we can catch it as soon as possible is ideal. This takes practice. Each time we do it the time shortens between the physical sensation signaling us and the emotional response pattern taking over. Initially, you might not realize this until after the re-action occurs. Perhaps, not even until the next day. This is normal. Still, take the time to playback what happened starting with the sensations you initially felt through the end of the interaction. Make the connection with your emotions, tend to whatever emotional needs you have, and breathe into the uncomfortable places in your body. For example, let's say you experience chronic lower back pain and you have identified that it is related to pent-up anger. You also are aware the pain flares up after interactions with your child. Let's create a scenario. You begin the day feeling great in your body. At a certain point, you have an interaction with your child that triggers you. You get angry and you do not express it. Suddenly your back seizes up. The pain draws your attention to a pattern of squashing your anger down, rather than expressing it in a healthy way. In this instance, your body is reminding you and inviting you to make a different choice. Ideally, you can take a moment to acknowledge the communication pattern, tend to the needs of the part of yourself connected with this pattern, then take mindful breaths into your back. There is an excellent chance the pain will subside. This repatterning through conscious awareness and action is what creates change.

The next time you find yourself in a similar situation making a different choice will be more accessible and hopefully, you will catch it before any symptoms occur. A different choice may look like taking a pause with your child by letting them know you are feeling frustrated (with the behavior not with them) and you need to step away, and then expressing the anger in a way that is not projected onto another such as movement, writing, chopping wood, kickboxing, or running. Or it may look like tending to your inner self that the pattern is related to. What do they need to not feel threatened? It is truly amazing what happens when we honor our emotions and listen to our bodies.

Here is a simple exercise to begin attuning to the felt sensations of your body and the emotions that accompany them.

EXERCISE

Tuning in With Your Emotions

Upon waking in the morning or before going to bed at night, take five minutes to sit quietly. Tune into your body and how you are feeling. This is an important beginning to taking care of your emotional body and deciphering your body's way of communicating.

1. Find a quiet place to sit, plant your feet firmly on the ground, and close your eyes. Begin to take gentle, rhythmic breaths.

2. Sense how you are feeling at that moment. Perhaps you can feel an emotion ready to burst forth that you have not given yourself the space to express. Perhaps you are not aware of anything in particular. That is ok. Stay present. We are always feeling something. Even "nothing" is something.

3. Now tune into your body. Are you sensing any areas of tightness and constriction? Perhaps your neck is sore, or your belly feels tight. Take note of where any areas of discomfort that are not related to recent physical exercise or trauma.

4. Pick one area and begin bringing your breath to that area. Allow the breath to soften this area. Ask yourself, "Is there anything to share about why I am feeling discomfort here?"

5. Perhaps you hear a response. Perhaps you experience an upwelling of emotion. Perhaps you feel tears brim to the surface or a scream that wants to be expressed. Perhaps you still do not feel anything, but you notice that directing your breath dissipates the tension.

6. Allow any emotional energy to move by simply continuing to breathe into it and express any emotions that arise. You will know you are complete when the discomfort subsides and you feel a lightness of being.

Acknowledging and expressing our emotional states is a crucial part of our evolution. If we are not willing to feel what is happening within us, our emotional responses and unmet needs can repeatedly sabotage us, causing a long trail of suffering. It also limits our capacity for experiencing emotions that feel incredible.

This exercise is a way to begin listening to the wisdom our body has to share. It is a start to being vulnerable in a way that is witnessed by our conscious selves. It is the beginning of accepting, loving, and welcoming all the parts of ourselves, even the ones lurking in the shadows that we are ashamed or scared of. Take the time to get acquainted with the vast spectrum of emotional states and discern the subtleties between them. Many of us have a limited emotional bandwidth containing a few "home" emotions. We are much more nuanced than we give ourselves credit for. One of the ways we can begin to expand our awareness is to expand our vocabulary of emotional descriptors. What are we really feeling?

Be specific. Below is a list to get started inspired by Dr. Bradley Nelson's list from his book, *The Emotion Code*.[5]

LIFESTYLE TIP

List of Emotional States

Sorrowful	Optimistic
Enraged	Eager
Tender	Empowered
Ecstatic	Joyful
Inspired	Free
Appreciative	Bitter
Awed	Betrayed
Vulnerable	Rejected
Apologetic	Unworthy
Enamored	Ashamed
Heartbroken	Insecure
Lost	Helpless
Passionate	Disgusted
Enthusiastic	Humiliated

Next time someone asks you how you are doing, rather than the mundane reply of "I'm good," try tuning into what you are really feeling and expressing it.

OUR WORST ENEMIES: GUILT & SHAME

Nothing puts the brakes on expressing how we are feeling faster than a good ol' dose of guilt and shame. This extends out to sharing our gifts with the world. Guilt and shame can be destroyers decimating any creation we attempt to put forth in a matter of seconds. Yet are they our worst enemies? It sure feels like it when the voices are running amok inside our heads. As we begin to recognize the circumstances that provoke our guilt and shame, we have an opportunity to gain awareness of old, wounded parts of ourselves.

Brené Brown defined shame in her most recent book, *Atlas of the Heart*, as "the intensely painful feeling or experience of believing that we are flawed and therefore unworthy of love, belonging, and connection."[6] In other words, a fundamental belief that "I am wrong." Guilt, on the other hand, is the belief that "I have done something wrong."

Often the parts of us that experience the deepest suffering are the parts associated with guilt and shame. They need to be approached with patience, tenderness, and loving curiosity. It may take time to coax these characters out of the shadows to develop a trusting relationship with them. However, it is time well spent. Our life is transformed as we learn to welcome the parts of ourselves that feel unworthy of love. The parts we are ashamed of are amongst those who feel the most unworthy. Learning to listen and love these parts is a process. Try getting curious and noticing when their voices emerge. It is most important to be gentle with ourselves in the discovery process.

DROPPING THE STORY

A significant barrier to completing an emotional response cycle is our attachment to the story. We unconsciously use narrative as a protective stance that positions us as victims. It keeps us disconnected from our bodies and hearts. Though we may experience feelings such as anger and fear when we are recycling a story, we inhibit the emotional response by focusing our attention on logical explanations versus on the felt sensation in our bodies. To better understand this, it is helpful to know that the words "feelings" and "emotions" that we frequently use interchangeably, have different meanings. Although there are variations in the definitions, the main distinction between the two is: emotions are based on instinct and sensation, whereas feelings are based on the stories we create around our emotional responses. These stories are derived from our past experiences.

It is easy to convince ourselves we are expressing our emotions as we toil over the way we were wronged by another. The irony is we are having feelings, *and* we are avoiding the uncomfortable sensations aroused by emotional responses by staying in the story. This loop could go on indefinitely without ever fully completing the emotional response cycle. When we hold on to a story, we interrupt the integration of the experience, instead stagnating the emotional energy flow. This stagnation contributes to pain, illness, and suffering. The next exercise gives you a chance to explore the difference between feelings and emotions, staying in the head and connecting with the body.

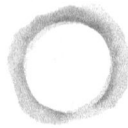

EXERCISE

What Am I Making This Mean?

Try playing with this exercise. Pay attention to how you feel compared to when you sit reeling in a story for hours, days, and sometimes even years.

1. Choose something minor that is currently happening in your life that you have feelings about, and you cannot seem to let go of the story of what happened.

2. Create an environment where you feel physically and emotionally safe to express yourself. If you are planning to throw things perhaps go outside. If you think you may want to scream, perhaps have pillows handy, music on, or request a time for the people you live with to be out of the house.

3. Be sure you schedule ample time to express. Sometimes you only need a few minutes, but other times once the box is opened, a cascade of emotions pours out.

4. When you are ready, let yourself begin connecting with the emotion that is readily available to you. If you have been thinking a lot about your situation, it is likely an emotion is readily available to tap into. If you have not been thinking about it, recall the situation that has been bothering you. Once you reconnect with the emotion(s), stop thinking about the story.

5. In some cases, the invitation alone is enough to start the flow of emotions. If this is true, ride the wave of all emotions that surface. They are like waves, so be sure to stay present long enough to allow different waves to roll in. Express until you feel complete.

6. If it is more challenging to drop the story and connect with the raw emotion, try asking yourself, "What am I making this mean?" Dig underneath the story to discover what it would mean about you or a belief you thought to be true if the story you had been telling yourself were the truth. For example, let's say your boss treated you horribly that day and "made you feel" like you were horrible at your job. You felt incredibly angry and kept thinking, "she is such a jerk." If you stay with this story, you have "anger" keeping you from what you are truly feeling. Do not be fooled that anger is all there is and that by you expressing anger you have completed the job. Ask yourself, "what am I making this mean?" By digging deeper, you may discover feelings of grief, shame, or unworthiness that you do not deserve this job or you are not smart enough to do it. Whatever thoughts arise, let yourself feel the emotions that come up as you dismantle the story by asking this powerful question.

7. If you find yourself returning to a narrative, continue to gently ask yourself what you are making it mean. Once you feel like you have detached from the story and felt all you can feel in that moment, complete the exercise with any self-soothing necessary. A good indicator that you are complete is no longer feeling a charge around the story and feeling in a lighter state than you felt before doing the exercise.

Some people spend the bulk of their lives angry with a person or a way they have been wronged. The only one that suffers here is the one attached to the story. Debilitating disease is birthed out of this. We must be willing to let the stories go. This exercise is fantastic for connecting with the emotions that we are truly feeling and often afraid to acknowledge. It is also a great tool for dismantling beliefs we have that are limiting us from accessing a much fuller spectrum of emotions.

SHAKE IT OFF

As I mentioned earlier in the chapter, by design we have an incredible capacity for "shaking off" traumatic experiences if only we would let ourselves do what is innate to our nervous systems. Our spines have a wave in them that supports trauma to move through our systems with grace and ease. As emotional energy becomes stagnant, the spinal wave is interrupted. Much like throwing boulders into a stream affects the flow of water, stuck emotional energy impacts the ability of the spine to facilitate resilience. Visionary Dr. Donny Epstein developed a brilliant body of work called *Network Spinal Analysis* that supports the body to release stagnant energy and revitalize this wave.[7] With our awareness, attention, breath, and intention, we can activate the spine to do its job and restore our greatest system of recovery.

Emotional expression also supports the process of trauma being able to move through us. When we let ourselves fully experience emotions as they arise, we also experience the relief and freedom in the moments afterward. As babies, we practiced this freedom of expression. We simply responded to our traumas. When hurt or scared, we would cry, shake, and move our bodies until we were complete. Sometimes there were waves of expression until the noticeable completion came with a sense of calm or a mood shift. As we had social rule upon social rule imposed upon us, we slowly began to stray from our innate ways and built protective walls around us. Our children can be great reminders of this. They are still connected to their instinctual selves. We need to return to this state of freedom of expression to allow ourselves to move toward optimum health. This is a fundamental practice for building self-trust. When we repeatedly send the message to ourselves that we are not worthy enough to honor our feelings, it chips away at our confidence. This has a severe impact on all areas of our lives. Repressing our emotions has massive implications including health problems, challenges setting boundaries, depression/sadness, grief, feeling lost, and more.

One of the most empowering choices we can make in our lives is to reconnect with our instincts. To do this, we need to be willing to feel the fullness of our emotions as they arise. This includes distressing emotions and joyful ones. Many of us have been shamed for feeling joy or pleasure as much as we have for expressing anger or tears. The pathway for doing this is to be present with the sensations in our bodies as our emotions arise. Be still, breathe, and ride the waves. This alone is a great accomplishment. For further healing, becoming acquainted with the parts of our inner selves and their needs steers us away from unhealthy patterns that cause illness toward a more vibrant life with a vast array of emotional experiences.

THREE

FEEDING OUR LIGHT BODY
– OUR DIETARY CHOICES

*The fact that our current planetary evolution is built
upon one creature having to physically consume
another to survive shows our deep limitation.*

RICHARD RUDD
Gene Keys

*Because there's no rule book for mystery illness,
there are also no limits to recovery.*

ANTHONY WILLIAMS

Every time we consume something, we have an opportunity to
feed our light body. What do I mean by the light body? Our
light body is our energetic body. It is within our physical body,
and it extends far beyond the borders of our physical body. It is
our chakra system, including our upper chakras, which exist outside of our physical bodies. When I refer to feeding the light body

in this chapter, I am referencing using food to support awakening higher states of consciousness. It means creating an environment (our bodies) that promotes vitality and purity.

WE ARE WHAT WE EAT

There is no denying that what we put into our bodies has a direct impact on our health and vitality. It can also be said that what we choose to eat has a direct impact on all the life forms we share this planet with. Let's have a short physics lesson. We know that everything is energy. Energy vibrates at different frequencies, faster vibrations equal higher frequencies and slower vibrations equal lower frequencies. Higher levels of consciousness equate to us vibrating at higher frequencies. If we consistently consume food that vibrates at a low frequency, this is going to have a direct impact on our vibrational rate. It can be deduced that eating high-quality food with a high vibrational state has a direct impact on the expansion of our consciousness.

Food can be used proactively to support awakening higher states of consciousness. It also provides a great reflection of our growth. For example, you may suddenly dislike a food that you have loved for a long time. Perhaps a food that always felt fine when you ate it previously, is now causing you digestive discomfort. In more extreme cases, your body may develop an intolerance or allergy to a food that for many years seemingly caused you no problem at all. These are excellent indicators that the food you are eating is no longer a good energetic match for you. For some people, the toxicity load in the body has become too high and their body is demanding a change. Either way, the toxicity levels, inflammatory nature, or perhaps simply the lack of nutrients in a food item, are no longer nourishing you in the way your body is demanding. You have outgrown that particular food and your body is requiring you to upgrade your diet to match the new energetic frequency you are being called to more fully embody. Listen to your body's wisdom. See it as a blessing and opportunity to become more vital, rather than a problem with your body.

Most food production today is not concerned with providing health and vitality to its consumers. On the contrary, its sole purpose seems to be profit over people. Many of us are aware at this point that many foods are poisoned with chemical additives, pesticides, hormones, and genetic modification. The factory-farming model of raising animals is disastrously unhealthy for the animals, the environment, and the consumer. Large-scale agriculture has depleted the soil of nutrients while replacing it with multiple toxic residues. There is ample documentation that shares the truth about how food is produced in our society today and the devastating effects it has on the Earth and our health. In addition to the more overt impact I have just stated, there are harmful physical, energetic, and emotional effects of consuming this quality of food, that are profound.

As with many things, the quality of food is not black and white. Processed foods, fast foods, and much of the food found in large chain supermarkets have little if any, vitality. There are many steps one can take from eating this type of food toward eating food that is as close to its original form as possible. For example, if you are not ready to stop eating meat altogether, you can stop eating cold cuts and fast food meat, or you can switch to organic meats that still come from large farms but are better for you because of what the animals are fed. Taking it a step further, you can raise animals for slaughter or buy from a local farm. This way you have full knowledge of what the animals consume and how they are treated. These are examples of steps in the right direction that have a higher quality than each prior example. You can also choose one meal a day to be plant-based or non-processed. Start slowly so that it feels easeful and not like a punishment. This is essential for lasting success. If it feels like you are restricting your diet, a mindset shift is required to emphasize the positive outcome of your choices. Sometimes making huge dietary changes can feel intimidating. Remember to be honest with yourself about where you are at, *without* self-judgment. Be gentle with yourself. Educate yourself about the many things that could be causing you to crave unhealthy foods. Anthony Williams' books are excellent references for this. Let making dietary changes feel empowering and inspiring, rather than be constricted or directed by others' opinions. See if you can get a friend or family member to join you and let it be a fun exploration of new foods.

LIFESTYLE TIP

One Meal a Day

It is amazing how beneficial eating one meal a day that is plant-based can have on our health and the health of the planet. We are faced with a serious crisis right now, on planet Earth, regarding climate change. The choices we make imminently have a profound effect on the success of all life on our planet. This time is unprecedented. It can be very overwhelming to think about and oftentimes we, as one person, feel we cannot make a difference. This is not true. We have a tremendous impact as individuals, and we also inspire others through our actions. Just like our bodies, the Earth knows how to heal itself. However, we humans must support the Earth's healing process by slowing down the rate of poisoning and magnitude of destruction we are doing so it can restore. Here are some facts for inspiration from Suzy Amis Cameron's book *The OMD Plan: Swap One Meal a Day to Save Your Health and Save the Planet.* [1]

- If you eat 1 plant-based meal a day for 1 year, you'll save almost 200,000 gallons of water (equal to 11,400 showers) *and* the pollution equivalent to 3,000 miles driven in a car.

- If everyone in the U.S. reduced their meat and dairy intake by just 50%, it would be equal to taking 26 million cars off the road.

- Eating plant-based reduces the risk of some cancers, supports a strong heart, reduces inflammation, reduces erectile dysfunction, lowers the risk of diabetes, and helps to maintain a healthy weight.

- Animal agriculture contributes more greenhouse gas than all transportation combined.

- Animal agriculture is the number one contributor to extinction and biodiversity loss due to land needed for grazing and growing feed.

- Livestock production is the largest contributor to global water pollution and a major driver of the ocean's 404 dead zones.

- Beef generates 20 times more greenhouse gas emissions and requires 20 times more land than beans per gram of protein.

Are you ready and willing to commit to eating one plant-based meal a day to support your health, as well as the health of our planet? This means no dairy products, eggs, fish, seafood, or meat. Ideally, it also means no processed, "fake" meat, or "fake" cheese products. If you decide to make this commitment, remember there are a whole host of highly processed, nutritionally deficient vegan foods on the market. Just because it is plant-based does not mean it is healthy. If you stick to foods that are closest to their natural state, you will have the most success at getting foods that are healthy for both your body and the planet.

WHAT IS HIGH VIBRATION FOOD ANYWAY?

Organic, biodynamic, plant-based foods that are in their closest form to how they grow naturally provide the highest quality of food. Conventional food production uses approximately 700 different insecticides, fungicides, and pesticides that negatively impact our health contributing to cancers, depression, and many other illnesses.[2] Although organic farming is not devoid of pesticide and fungicide use, there are parameters that make it significantly better for the Earth and our bodies. A recent study found that switching to an organic diet reduced the cancer-causing herbicide glyphosate found in the most used herbicide, Monsanto's Round-up, in the participants' bodies by 70% in just three days.[3] Additionally, factory-farmed animals are given antibiotics, leading to antibiotic-resistant bacteria which we also are exposed to upon consumption. Transitioning to an organic diet relieves us of exposure to a multitude of toxic substances that have been shown to contribute to illness.

Biodynamic farming has an even more harmonious relationship with the Earth than organic farming. In addition to being organic, it takes into consideration the cycles of the seasons, the moon, and what type of plants grow best in different cyclical conditions. It adds a spiritual layer to farming by growing with the rhythms of the Earth. It honors the interconnected relationship between the land, the plants, the farmers, and the cosmos with a heightened emphasis on sustainability for all.

Having access to this quality of food can be challenging for a variety of reasons. Many areas simply do not have stores nearby that sell organic produce. In low-income areas, sometimes the only place to buy food is convenience stores. Fresh produce does not have a long shelf life; therefore, stores will frequently opt for items that will last longer. There are non-profit groups working to bring healthier foods and more variety to areas that are "food deserts," as well as financial support from benefit programs that give participants more buying power.[4] The availability of organic foods is becoming greater each year because of increasing demand. If you do not have access to high-quality food because of finances or availability, there are some options such as growing your own food, joining a local CSA (community-supported agriculture) farm, participating in a community garden plot or food bank, or using a delivery service.

Fortunately, there is a wide range of qualities between organic, biodynamic food and those that are artificial and harmful. For example, if most of your diet consists of highly processed foods, incorporating more fresh, non-organic fruits and vegetables is a huge step in a healthier direction. Each of us can assess where we are at and see what steps we can take toward a healthier diet. Every step is progress, and the benefits are not to be underestimated. Let's take an even closer look at why organic, plant-based foods can have higher vitality. Perhaps with additional understanding, the need to prioritize healthier food will become increasingly clear.

It is important to grasp that we cannot consume other life forms that have suffered and have been treated poorly without this having a direct impact on our state of vitality. Pause, take a breath, and read that sentence again. I believe when we reach a certain state of consciousness, we will no longer have the desire to eat another

> It is important to grasp that we cannot consume other life forms that have suffered and have been treated poorly without this having a direct impact on our state of vitality.

animal to feed ourselves. We also would not consider eating a vegetable that is modified and covered in toxic chemicals. Not only would we not feel well, but it would also not make logical sense to do this. As we learn to listen more deeply to our bodies, our tolerance for consciously ingesting toxic things diminishes. We will gravitate toward foods that allow us to feel energized, strong, light, and alive. As we apply one aspect of the *Wheel of Whole Body Healing* to our lives and gain a new understanding of ourselves, we will hear other aspects beckoning for attention. Making dietary changes is one of the easiest and fastest ways to yield palpable results. Although we can have emotional ties to food, our diet is habituation. Oftentimes, if we make a new choice and stick to it for a few weeks, the cravings will subside. If they do not subside, look at how balanced your diet is to be sure you are getting all the essential building blocks needed to thrive and adjust/supplement as needed. Shifting to higher quality, nutrient-dense food is worth it, on every level.

Ultimately, we must strive to make choices that serve life rather than take from it. When we consume animals from a dissociated, dishonoring place or eat food that is toxic to us, we are not choosing life. We cannot *fully* thrive in this choice. We see the results of that very clearly in our world today. Greedy choices regarding food production have caused great degradation to the land and animals. The results of these choices are a population of people that are staggeringly unhealthy and suffering, as well as a planet that is threatened by the mass extinction of many species. We are dealing with pollution and toxicity on a massive scale and our bodies are suffering from this. What we consume is a huge way to take our power back, take responsibility for our health, and be responsible citizens of Earth. The great news is food can be ultra-healthy, high-vibration, and super tasty too.

LIFESTYLE TIP

Recipes

Below I have included some delicious recipes from my cookbook, *FOOD for the light body - simple plant-based & gluten-free recipes for the body & soul.*[5] There is a recipe for each season, though they can be enjoyed in any season. Let them inspire you to eat a nourishing, clean, high-vibration meal that will support your health and consciousness while satiating your palate as well.

SPRING

Tuscan Tempeh
4 servings

Ingredients:

Tempeh:
2 tablespoons olive oil
2 blocks of original / plain tempeh, cubed into bite-sized pieces
½ teaspoon brown mustard seeds
1 bulb of fennel, feathery tops only, chopped
2 large tomatoes, diced
½ teaspoon Real salt
¼ teaspoon black pepper
zest of whole lemon
1 teaspoon maple syrup
2 teaspoons fresh rosemary, chopped

Mixed Vegetables:
2 cups broccoli florets, 1 fennel bulb, sliced, 1 bunch
    asparagus, cut into bite-sized pieces, and 4
    leaves green kale (or any veggies you like)
1 large clove of garlic, chopped
½ teaspoon Real salt
1 tablespoon lemon juice

Carmelized Onions:
1 teaspoon olive oil
1 small yellow onion, sliced thinly into half moons
2 teaspoons apple cider vinegar (balsamic works well too)
½ teaspoon molasses (maple syrup also works well)

Preparation:

For the tempeh:

1. Heat olive oil in a non-stick pan on medium heat. Add the tempeh and mustard seeds, and cook for 8-10 minutes, stirring until they are lightly browned. If the tempeh is burning try turning down the heat a little or add a little more olive oil.

2. Add remaining ingredients and turn down the heat to medium-low. Cook until the tomatoes reduce into more of a sauce. Salt and pepper to taste and set aside.

For the mixed vegetables:

1. In a non-stick pan, sauté vegetables on medium heat in olive oil until desired tenderness. Veggies can be steamed as an alternative.

2. Once they are done cooking, turn off the heat and season with the juice of half a lemon. Salt and pepper to taste.

For the caramelized onions:

1. Sauté onion in olive oil until glassy (2-3 minutes).

2. Just before turning off the heat, add vinegar and molasses and stir well. Be sure to turn on the stove fan before adding vinegar! Cook for a couple more minutes until the liquid is reduced and the onions are caramelized. Set aside.

To assemble:

Make a pile of the vegetables on each plate. Beautifully arrange the tempeh and sauce on top of the veggie base. Top the dish with small pile of caramelized onions and a sprig of fresh rosemary.

SUMMER

Romaine Leaf Tacos with Sundried Tomato Paté, Lacinato Kale, & Blue Potatoes
3-4 servings

We LOVE these tacos. This is a great recipe for improvising with the ingredients you have in the refrigerator.

Ingredients:

Sundried Tomato Paté:
1 small clove of garlic
6 oil-packed sundried tomatoes, rinsed in hot water
½ cup raw sunflower seeds
1 tablespoon olive oil
½ teaspoon Real salt

Taco filling:
2 tablespoons olive oil
3 cups blue potatoes, diced (any kind
   of potato can be substituted)
3 cups lacinato kale, thinly sliced
1 ripe avocado
romaine lettuce leaf

Cashew-Jalapeño Cream:
¾ cup raw cashews
a very thin slice of jalapeño (ancho pepper works well too)
¼ teaspoon of Real salt
½ cup water

Preparation:

For the Cashew Cream:
Blend all the ingredients in a high-speed blender on high, for approximately 1 minute, until the sauce is creamy. You may need to scrape the sides down a few times. Be sure to start with a small slice of spicy pepper. I have made the mistake of adding too big a piece and it was very spicy. You can always add more. Add salt and pepper to taste. Consistency should be thick but pour easily out of the blender. This sauce keeps well, refrigerated, in a sealed container for 2 days.

For the Paté:
Blend the garlic in a food processor. Add remaining ingredients and blend for 1 minute. Scrape down the sides and blend for another minute.

For the tacos:
Heat the olive oil in a medium, non-stick pan on medium heat. Add the potatoes and some salt and stir well. First, let the potatoes brown a little bit, and then add enough water to cover the bottom of the pan. Cover the potatoes and let them steam until the water runs out. If the potatoes are still hard when the water evaporates, repeat this step. Once they are soft, add the kale and stir well. You may want to add a little more olive oil at this point if the potatoes are sticking. Cook for a few minutes until the kale softens. Remove from the heat.

To assemble:
Place two big romaine leaves on each plate. Divide the sundried tomato paté equally between each taco and distribute it evenly along the spine of the leaf. This paté is packed with flavor so you do not need to put very much in each one. Next, scoop the potato mixture into each taco. Top the potatoes with thin slices of avocado. Lastly, top the tacos with cashew-jalapeño sauce.

AUTUMN

Purple Top Turnip Thai Coconut Curry
4 servings

Ingredients:
1 tablespoon coconut oil
⅓ cup yellow onion, finely diced
2 cloves of garlic, minced
1 inch of fresh ginger root, finely grated
1 small red bell pepper, diced
2 cups butternut squash, peeled and cut into bite-sized
   cubes (pie pumpkin or sweet potato can also be used)
1 cup cauliflower, cut into bite-sized florets
1 carrot, sliced into half-moons
1 large purple top turnip, unpeeled, cut into bite-sized cubes
1 teaspoon jalapeño (or spicy pepper of your choice) finely diced
a 15 oz. can of full-fat coconut milk
1 cup water
2-3 kaffir lime leaves
2 teaspoons Real salt
2 leaves of swiss chard or green kale, thinly sliced
½ lime, juiced

Preparation:

1. Melt coconut oil in a soup pot on medium heat. Add onion and cook for 1-2 minutes until glassy.

2. Add garlic, ginger, and bell pepper; cook for a few more minutes to blend flavors. Add remaining veggies except for greens and stir well. Add coconut milk, water, kaffir lime leaves, and salt. Cover and cook until vegetables are tender but not so tender they fall apart (15-20 min).

3. Remove from heat and stir in the greens and lime juice. Salt to taste. Serve over a bed of black forbidden rice or jasmine rice. Remember to remove the kaffir lime leaves before serving. They are not for eating and are a choking hazard.

WINTER

Portuguese Kale Soup
4 servings

This brothy soup is very warming on a cold day. I like to use chipotle pepper because the smoky flavor resembles the traditional flavor of this soup. You can also use cayenne if you cannot find chipotle powder. Cayenne is spicier; therefore, I recommend starting with 1/4 teaspoon and working your way up to the heat level you prefer.

Ingredients:
1 cup yellow onion, diced
2 tablespoons olive oil
2 cloves of garlic, minced
1½ teaspoons dried thyme
2 medium carrots, sliced into half-moons
2 medium potatoes, diced into small pieces
   (Yukon gold preferred, but any will work)
2 cups cooked red kidney beans (or a 15 oz. can)
2 tomatoes, diced (or 1 - 15 oz. can of
   diced tomatoes with liquid)
2½ teaspoons Real salt
5 cups water
½ teaspoon chipotle powder (for a mild spice level)
4 cups packed green curly kale, leaves and stems, thinly sliced
¼ cup packed fresh parsley, leaves & stems, chopped
¼ of lemon

Preparation:

1. Sauté the onion in olive oil in a medium soup pot. After a couple of minutes, add the garlic and thyme.

2. Add carrots and potatoes and sauté for 2 more minutes. Add kidney beans, tomatoes, salt, water, and chipotle. Stir well, cover, and turn the heat up to high.

3. Once the soup is boiling, reduce to medium heat and cook until potatoes are tender, approximately 15 minutes.

4. Stir in the kale and cook for a minute more before taking it off the heat. Add salt and chipotle pepper to taste. Garnish each bowl with a good portion of fresh parsley and a squeeze of lemon juice. Serve immediately.

FOUR

PHYSICAL AILMENTS & IMBALANCES

Diseases are healed- not by using the Spiritual to heal the physical, not by using willpower to force others to conform to your way of thinking, not by the application of brute force, but by the uncovering of the Perfection that is already there.

DR. ROBERT A. RUSSELL

AN ALTERNATIVE APPROACH TO ILLNESS

Disempowerment manifests in the physical body in every way imaginable. What I mean by disempowerment is our unspoken truths, our unexpressed emotions, our disconnection from source energy, our habit of staying in patterns that keep us small, and our lack of self-love. When we stay in states of disempowerment over periods of time, the energetic ripple begins to swell and manifests in our physical bodies in the form of aches, pains, and disease. I believe that physical imbalances that we experience begin in our energy fields as a form of disempowerment.

Our bodies have the incredible power, by design, to heal themselves. Part of our job in supporting this innate ability is to listen to what our bodies are telling us and take the necessary actions to facilitate healing. There is not one prescribed message for everyone with the same symptoms. Each individual has a complex and unique set of circumstances. This is why learning how to listen to our bodies (rather than have another person tell us what we need) is extremely important skill for healing. Luna's Story is an example of deep listening. During a session, the message she received was to reclaim her body as her own sovereign space. Her immediate willingness to command absolute reclamation dissolved the remaining Lyme disease symptoms.

Luna's Story – Lyme Disease

Some years ago, the renowned healer Charlie Goldsmith[1] put out a call for energy healers worldwide to submit applications to be part of a team of healers. At the time, he was collaborating with researchers so they could better understand how energy healing radically altered a person's experience of pain within minutes. I was excited to be a part of this movement of investigative inquiry as I knew firsthand the power energy healing had to effectively serve people. I invited Luna to have her case be shared as part of this application. She had been diagnosed with Lyme disease two years prior. At that time, she had done a variety of treatments to address the symptoms, which had become extreme. When she came to me, her symptoms were not as severe as her worst moments, but she still had intense joint pain, fatigue, and digestive problems.

After just one session, Luna's joint pain was gone. She was able to do yoga for the first time in two years and she was pain-free. She felt vital and inspired. She began doing meditation and her spiritual practices again. Her digestion was significantly better and improving with each day.

During this session, Luna experienced a warm, tingling sensation (healing energy) washing over her body and a more potent connection with her higher self than she had ever felt before. She received instructions from her higher self on how to facilitate healing. She was invited to reclaim the temple of her body and declare the Lyme consciousness to leave right now. When she did this, she received a huge rush of healing energy, deepening her connection with her will power. Following up with Luna three months later, she was still completely pain-free. Her digestive symptoms that had persisted immediately after the session took a few weeks to subside, progressively improving as each day passed. During her session, Luna was a receptive listener to her inner guidance. She heard the message and immediately acted on it without hesitation or doubt.

Every person is capable of sensing guidance from their higher selves. In Luna's case, she was guided to reclaim her body as her temple. Others with similar symptoms may be guided to do something completely different. The important message of Luna's story is not reclaiming the body to neutralize the symptoms (that guidance came from within her, for her,) but rather that *listening to the wisdom that comes from within you can be extremely beneficial when navigating symptoms.* Following is an exercise for developing your inner listening skills by getting curious about your pain.

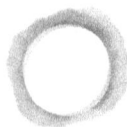

EXERCISE

Listening to Your Pain

This is an exercise to introduce opening to your pain, rather than a more common response of resisting it or wanting to make it disappear. When you get curious about what your pain is trying to communicate, a wealth of awareness about yourself becomes available. (An exercise to practice Connecting to Your Higher Self & Spirit Guides is in chapter 6.)

1. Find a comfortable position. Close your eyes and bring your attention to your breath. Allow your breath to be deep and relaxed.

2. When you are ready, bring your attention to a place of physical pain in your body.

3. With your intention, bring your breath to this place. Let your breath bathe this area in acceptance and love.

4. Now comes the fun part. Get curious about what your body is trying to communicate with you via this pain. Some examples to explore are: Are you pushing yourself? Are you avoiding speaking your truth about something? Are you resisting a change that you know you need to make in an area of life? Are you giving your power away to another? Are you eating something you know is not healthy for you? Are you hesitant to forgive yourself or another?

5. Ask the painful part of your body if it wants to communicate anything with you. Ask what it needs to feel supported.

6. Try to have an open mind and let the answers flow freely, without judgment. The answers may come to you in the form of words, a feeling/knowing, an image, a sound, or something else. Whatever information comes your way, observe it, as is, without placing extra meaning on it by trying to logically make sense of it. If you sense that an inner self is residing in the place of pain, you may want to shift to the Dialoguing with Your Inner Selves exercise in Chapter 2 at this point.

7. Repeat this practice, especially if you have chronic pain. By doing it, you are giving your body the message that you are ready and willing to listen. Sometimes it takes time and space to open especially when we have silenced ourselves for a long time.

One of the powerful things about listening is that we are guided through accumulated layers of resistance toward the root of an imbalance. Sometimes it is clear immediately, upon tuning into the body, what the root cause is. Other times, it requires moving through different layers and addressing the needs that arise before the root presents itself. It is essential to uncover and address the energetic root of a physical imbalance to allow lasting healing to transpire. If the root is not addressed, and only the physical symptoms are, reoccurrence can happen.

. . .

When my daughter was two weeks old, she began to show signs of thrush. I was pretty sure the white on her tongue was not just milk residue. Part of me did not want it to be true, so I fell into a longstanding avoidance pattern instead of addressing it. Four weeks later, the thrush had progressed and needed to be addressed. During my meditation one morning, I had so much self-judgment coming up (another longstanding pattern of mine) for not having listened to myself and dealt with it sooner. As tears of frustration fell, an opportunity presented itself. At that moment, I decided to forgive myself for the choice I had made, along with the past choices I had made, to ignore my body when symptoms arose. Suddenly, I experienced a release of energy. As I was willing to meet my pain with gentleness and love, a flood of resources became available to me. I could see a way to relieve my daughter's thrush that I could not see before. From this place of new receptivity, I was able to employ the resources I had available. I gave her a healing session and applied the wisdom of the *Wheel*. During the session, it was revealed that I had layers of unexpressed emotions that were contributing to her susceptibility to thrush. I shifted my attention to being present with these emotions of unworthiness and anger by acknowledging and expressing them. Over the next few days, the thrush quickly subsided. In this case, the root cause was related to my unexpressed emotional energy. As I addressed this, the energetic influence my unexpressed emotions had shifted, and my daughter's body biome reorganized to a state of more balance and optimum health.

> It is essential to uncover and address the energetic root of a physical imbalance to allow lasting healing to transpire.

Eli's story is another example of how addressing the root allowed rapid shifts in his physical experience to occur. In his case, there was also a build-up of emotional energy causing physical symptoms. Once we discovered and addressed the cause, we took it one step further and implemented a plan to prevent overwhelm.

Eli's Story – Mysterious Body Pains

Eli came to me because he was experiencing pain radiating all over his body. It seemed to come from out of nowhere and was not going away. He scheduled a time to go see the doctor and was referred to me a few days before his appointment. In our session, we discovered that he was holding a lot of unexpressed grief plus shame and guilt. We attended to this accumulation of emotional energy in his energy field first, followed by the invitation to let the emotional energy move through breath, movement, and expression. Lastly, we invited love to wash over and inhabit his whole body. By the end of the session, Eli was feeling a profound lightness of being with the sensation of pain noticeably reduced.

Over the next few days, the pain in his body completely dissolved. By the time he went to the doctor, the pain was gone. He followed through with the recommended tests anyways and the results came back healthy and normal.

During Eli's session, we discovered it was important for him to learn how to prevent his emotions, as well as those of others, from accumulating in his energy field. I taught him a simple grounding exercise to be done as a daily habit to tend to his energy field. In time, he noticed that when he practiced tending to his energy field with consistency, he felt great. When he neglected to do this for a few consecutive days, he would feel hints of pain returning.

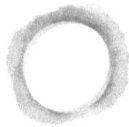

EXERCISE

Grounding Emotional Energy

This is a simple and important practice of self-care. I invite you to approach this practice as a daily prayer.

1. Find a place outside, ideally a place that is quiet where you can have your bare feet on the earth. If you are in a city, no worries. Choose a spot where you feel connected with the Earth.

2. Close your eyes and feel imaginary roots growing out of the soles of your feet down deep into the Earth.

3. Imagine anything that is not serving your highest good being released through the soles of your feet and feeding the soil beneath you.

4. When you are ready, visualize every cell in your body being filled with the love of Mother Earth. Feel it rising through the soles of your feet and circulating around your whole body. Take the time to imagine the smallest particles that make up the physical you, all the way out to the farthest reaches of your energy field.

5. Spend at least a few minutes letting yourself be nourished by Mother Earth. You will know you are complete when you feel more centered and grounded in yourself. More

psychic space has now been created for you to move throughout your day with ease.

This grounding practice only takes a few moments to do and makes a huge difference. You will experience more happiness and less overwhelm by making this a regular part of your day. To learn more about the benefits of grounding, check out the book *Earthing*.[2] This simple practice has exceptional benefits for our health and is something readily available to us that we often take for granted.

...

Oftentimes, throughout the journey of peeling back layers to the root, we become aware of unconscious patterns that are a fundamental part of the cause. In this case, it is crucial to get clear on exactly what the pattern is and create a new plan that can be put into practice whenever the old pattern kicks in. Having awareness and taking new action are key elements for success and lasting change. It can be difficult to do this on our own. Having skilled professional guidance such as a psychotherapist or an expert life coach is irreplaceable when it comes to seeing our unconscious patterns more clearly.

Sometimes the root cause can be tricky to determine. Fortunately, it is not necessarily essential to know the root from the onset. We can begin by applying the *Wheel* to initiate exploration. Throughout this process, deeper layers will likely reveal themselves that point toward the bedrock of discomfort. In Alyssa's Story, the key lessons she gained from her session focused on chronic sinus problems were *how to build her confidence, to know she had options*, and that *she can choose what feels aligned for her and have a successful outcome.*

Alyssa's Story – Chronic Sinus Problems

Alyssa and I had already been working together when she shared that ever since she was a child, she had sinus issues. She consistently had trouble sleeping because she couldn't breathe out of her nose. She also suffered from allergies and a lot of sneezing. Recently, the doctor suggested she get surgery to remedy the problem. Alyssa was not interested in surgery or prescription medications if they could be avoided, so she held off on that recommendation.

In the evening, after we did our session, Alyssa's situation flared up and she had great difficulty breathing. The following day she felt a big improvement. She was feeling less allergic and sneezing much less. She was able to meditate for the first time without mouth breathing. This allowed her to settle into a deeper state of relaxation. She also had the same experience with sleeping that night. For the next several days, her sinuses felt more open each day. This continued until the symptoms subsided.

Ultimately, she did not need to seek surgical intervention or medication. Though we did not come to any clear conclusions about root causes in this session, so much movement happened simply by her making an empowered choice to be present with her symptoms and open to receiving love.

It is common that mystery symptoms traditional medicine cannot pinpoint are caused by energetic imbalances. Physical symptoms have an energetic blueprint as the foundation of their physical expression. We are energetic beings. Everything affects us. Some things cause energetic waves (or tsunamis) that when not dealt with can become physical symptoms. This is especially true when we have long-term exposure to the "wave." Examples of common "waves" are trauma, emotional upset, substance use/abuse, grief and loss, viruses, chemical exposure, negative communication patterns, co-dependent relationships, poor boundaries, and unhealthy diets. In some instances, as we learn to listen more subtly to the cues our body is sending, there is the opportunity to make lifestyle changes before physical symptoms arrive.

Fret not if a symptom is not caught in these early stages, there are innumerable steps along the way for healing and growth. One of the keys is to become curious about our symptoms/condition. In our curiosity, we can hear the wisdom of our bodies, explore beliefs we may be harboring about our condition, and learn how to be loving and kind to ourselves. With curiosity, we can learn to accept and celebrate who we are, moment to moment. This is the true nature of healing. Sometimes healing equates with a cure and oftentimes it is about something much more all-encompassing that we can begin to catch a glimpse of with curiosity.

> Sometimes healing equates with a cure and oftentimes it is about something much more all-encompassing that we can begin to catch a glimpse of with curiosity.

In Laura's Story, you will see how her curiosity about her thyroid cancer and her appreciation of her thyroid had a powerful impact on her original diagnosis.

Laura's Story – Thyroid Cancer

Laura is a naturopathic doctor and a colleague who was diagnosed with an aggressive form of thyroid cancer. Her response to this diagnosis was inspiring. Instead of being overwhelmed with the fear of having cancer, she chose to appreciate her thyroid for the many years of healthy functioning it provided her. She interacted with her cancer cells, concluding that they were not wrong or bad, but rather confused cells. She even celebrated her thyroid with a farewell party before she had surgery to remove it.

Just before her surgery, Laura graciously accepted my offering of a session to support her healing process. Until that point, she had turned down many healers because they were "making the cancer wrong and trying to get rid of it." She saw her cancer as a gift bearing many important messages for her and I shared this perspective. During the session, we went to a very deep place that involved the invitation for her to use her voice in a more active and empowered way in her life. This was tied to many patterns from early on that had repeated throughout the years. I became aware that if she chose to, she could heal her thyroid completely without surgery.

A few days later, Laura decided to follow through with the surgery to remove her thyroid. When they came back with the post-surgery results, the doctor shared the tumor had shrunk to three times smaller than a few weeks prior when she received her biopsy results, and that the cancer was now a non-aggressive form. Laura's choice to appreciate and celebrate her thyroid, to not reject the cancer as something bad, and our session were powerful remedies for supporting her body to heal itself. The following exercise is an opportunity to cultivate curiosity about your pain. This may be a very different approach to your body, condition, and pain than you have taken before. The only thing required is to do your best at being curious and open.

EXERCISE

Breathing Love into Your Pain

Let Laura's story be an inspiration for this exercise. If you are experiencing physical pain, explore this breathing exercise and see what happens. Try to remain open to the possibility that your pain can subside. We need to believe we can heal to allow ourselves to heal. Let this exercise stretch your view of what is possible.

1. Choose a place that is peaceful where you can relax as much as possible.

2. Allow your breath to deepen as much as you can while remaining relaxed. Take gentle inhalations and exhalations through either your mouth or nose.

3. Tune in with the story you have regarding a particular pain. Do you find yourself hating it, wishing it would go away? Are you blaming it for ruining your quality of life? Do your thoughts harbor words of rejection, disassociation, abandonment, or fear? Be honest about the story you tell yourself about your pain.

4. Now place your hands gently on the location of your pain.

5. Begin to focus your breath on this location. You may be able to physically feel the breath move this part of your

body, or you may not, depending on where it is. Either way, use your intention to bring your breath to this place.

6. Spend a couple of minutes breathing into your pain.

7. When you are ready, begin appreciating this part of your body. If you find this challenging because it has caused you so much pain, begin by appreciating your body as a whole for being a vessel to have this experience called life.

8. Complete this exercise after at least a few minutes of focused breathing and appreciation. Notice how you feel as you open your eyes. Has the quality of the sensation changed in any way? Have the stories in your head shifted in relation to your pain?

9. Repeat this practice with consistency and frequency.

When our mind becomes a tireless cheerleader for our body's innate healing ability, we can access an infinite well of possibility. As we begin to listen to what our body tells us about its imbalances, and we have the courage to look deeper at what our aches and pains represent, we can experience just how magnificent we are in our unstoppable ability to heal.

FIVE

OUR ENERGY FIELDS

Absence of evidence is not evidence of their absence.

UNKNOWN

Our energetic presence is vast. It reaches far beyond the confines of the physical body. Sometimes, the cause of symptoms in the physical body is imbalances in the energy field. Medicine people from indigenous tribes have known this for ages. Their work is done in the unseen realms, in the place where everything and anything is possible. Traditional medicine systems, such as Chinese medicine (e.g. acupuncture) and Ayurvedic medicine, are built upon meridians (flowing rivers of energy contained within our bodies) and chakras (energy centers within and above the body). Just because conventional medicine does not share this perspective, it does not mean it does not exist or is irrelevant. As a practitioner, this was one of the primary terrains I worked within to support healing.

BIOFIELD SCIENCE

The definition of the biofield is evolving as scientists continue to grasp its vastness. The development of the field of psychoneuroimmunology validated for Western scientists and researchers that all the systems of the body communicate with one another within the container of one larger system. This exploration led to the next question, "how big is this system?" Dr. Shamini Jain discussed the nature of the biofield in her book, *Healing Ourselves: Biofield Science and the Future of Health.*[1] Dr. Jain stated biofields are "sets of interpenetrating and interacting fields of energy and information – some of them dense and electromagnetic in nature and some more subtle in nature."[2] Biofield research pioneer Dr. Beverly Rubik and colleagues discussed the biofield as being an organizing principle that "can influence and be influenced by a variety of biological pathways including biochemical, cellular, and neurological processes as they modulate activity and information flow across multiple levels of living systems."[3] The biofield's nature is electromagnetic *and* quantum affecting the smallest individual particles to massive planetary movements.

In lay terms, this can be translated as every living thing has an energy field within and surrounding it. This energy field is a container for our physical, emotional, sexual, and spiritual responses. It is alive and interactive. Simply put, it means that every thought, action, etc. affects everything. We are interconnected to all aspects of ourselves, *and* we are interconnected with all that is alive. This means the biofield can be used to transmit information to systems in the physical body. Distance healing is an example of this. It is what enables practitioners like myself to do healing sessions for someone on the other side of the globe without ever seeing their face. When we learn how to communicate within the biofield, the prospects for healing become very different.

Nearly two decades ago, one of my spiritual mentors, Drunvalo Melchizedek, introduced me to the electromagnetic, toroidal field that surrounds our hearts. He devised a meditation practice that included sensing these fields and how they exist within a larger toroidal field that surrounds each of us.[4] I spent several years exploring this practice. It helped me develop skills working in my outer energy field.

In 2004, the Director of Research at the HeartMath Institute, Rollin McCraty, wrote a scientific paper that shared how the heart has a large, toroidal-shaped electromagnetic field that interacts with other hearts' electromagnetic fields when in proximity.[5] It revealed the intelligence of how our hearts communicate with all our cells, as well as how our hearts communicate with other living beings through their electromagnetic fields.

For example, the energy field around our hearts responds to the thoughts and emotions we are having. When another person is in proximity to us, our thoughts and emotions will be communicated to and affect their heart's energy field whether either is aware of it or not. This introduces an important concept called coherence.

> When another person is in proximity to us, our thoughts and emotions will be communicated to and affect their heart's energy field whether either is aware of it or not.

Coherence is the synchronization of rhythmic activities in living systems.[6] It happens when "the heart, brain, autonomic nervous system, immune system, endocrine system, thoughts, and emotions are in alignment."[7] This is relevant because when we are in coherence, we are functioning in a more optimum state of health. Many things disrupt coherence such as stress. The Heart-Math Institute has continued researching our magnificent hearts and developing user-friendly technology to monitor coherence, as well as transforming hospital cultures with their research and technology.[8] The next exercise will help you sense your toroidal field and return to a state of coherence.

EXERCISE

Sensing Your Heart's Toroidal Field

If you can, visit the HeathMath website to see an image of the toroidal field surrounding the heart[9]. At the very least look up what a toroidal shape is so you have a sense of it. It is a doughnut shape with the heart residing in the center "hole" and the energy field leaving and returning to the heart in a spherical, spiral-like manner. There are also computer-generated videos that show the direction of the energy flow.

This exercise will focus on sensing the heart's electromagnetic field. If you wish to further this practice, you can explore sensing the much larger toroidal field that Drunvalo Melchizedek said extends 65 feet above and below the head. This is excellent practice for developing subtle listening skills.

1. Find a comfortable seat in a quiet space.

2. Take some moments to quiet your mind and connect with your breath.

3. When you are ready, turn your attention to your heart center in the middle of your chest. Begin by observing if you notice anything. Do you sense movement? Do you see the field with your inner eye? If you do, skip the remaining steps, and simply revel in the incredulous nature of the heart.

4. Pull up the image of the toroidal field around your heart in your mind's eye. Use your imagination to see it there. It is there, even if you may not be able to sense it at first. To begin developing sensitivity to it, imagine it.

5. If you could sense it, what does it look like, feel like, or sound like? Give yourself the freedom to set aside any doubts by accepting it exists and move on to sensing.

6. Stay in this state of subtle observation for as long as you like.

It may take time to begin sensing the heart's toroidal field. One thing I can say is that sensing comes in many forms. Try not to doubt what is revealed to you. It is easy to think you felt something and then immediately dismiss it as nothing. It took me several weeks of practice when I first started this to begin feeling what was happening. With patience, something pertinent will be revealed.

LOVING VS. RELEASING

There is a lot of talk in the "spiritual self-help" world about releasing energetic cords and "negative" energy from our bodies and energy fields. For years, I also put this concept into practice. It took me a long time to realize when I was releasing something there was a myriad of beliefs that were not moving me toward my goal of wellness and freedom. For example, when oriented toward releasing, our attention is focused on what we do not want rather than what we do want. This will likely create a never-ending loop of things to release. For me, there were times an avoidance pattern was at play. Releasing became a way of not needing to be present with the uncomfortable feelings I had or the parts I was ashamed of. Instead, I was spiritually bypassing, convincing myself I was dealing with something, when I was not at all. When there are parts of ourselves that we are "releasing", we are in turn rejecting ourselves. Instead, we need to provide compassion, forgiveness, and love; they are a part of us. Perhaps the most significant revelation I had was recognizing that releasing is often based on fear rather than love.

Sometimes we are susceptible to being influenced by unwanted energies (energies other than ourselves). When this is the case, fortifying our energy fields by bringing more love to the parts of ourselves vulnerable to unwanted energies creates a natural repellent. Similarly, love and compassion are necessary anchors when inviting unwanted energies to leave our energy field. Like a parent to a child, when we face a frightened child with steadfast love, the child will likely follow our guidance. The same holds true for unwanted energies. If you suspect there are entities you are hosting in your energy field, it is best to contact someone who has experience with sending them home. I encourage you to use great discernment when choosing a practitioner who works in the unseen realms. Trust your instincts and if something feels off, speak up or leave. The intention of sharing this information is not to encourage you to direct unwanted energies on your own without skills/guidance, but rather to understand the difference between orienting toward love rather than releasing as fortification for our energy fields.

> When we have repulsion or a "getting rid of" attitude, especially if it is related to a challenging relationship or life experience, we neglect to honor the reciprocity of our life events contributing to who we are today.

As humans that are interconnected, we are not infallible. As part of my evening meditation practice, I regularly ask my guides to cleanse my field of anything not serving my highest good. I also use releasing techniques for specific conditions frequently related to pathogens causing physical illness. The difference is lovingly letting go of that which no longer serves us with an appreciation for ourselves, the other, and all that it has taught us. When we have repulsion or a "getting rid of" attitude, especially if it is related to a challenging relationship or life experience, we neglect to honor the reciprocity of our life events contributing to who we are today. We are the sum of all our experiences. Our life experience is what best prepares us to serve others with sincerity. This includes the difficult experiences we have weathered. By walking the path of our lives, we cultivate compassion for others who have had similar experiences. Our suffering is part of what connects us. When we live our lives embracing all of who we are, our suffering included, we become compassionate leaders guiding our communities. It fuels our purpose.

A way to shift away from releasing (fearing) toward loving is to visualize our energy fields filled with love. This may look like a white or golden light or feel like a warm liquid washing through and around you. Even if you use releasing, let it not be the focus for balancing your energy field. Remember, where we place our attention is where the energy flows. Spending time basking in golden, healing light will serve you more than repetitively releasing and removing the "other" from your energy field. This coupled with other exercises such as boundary setting (chapter 8) and dialoguing with your inner selves (chapter 2) provides a solid approach for maintaining a well-balanced energy field.

EXERCISE

Activating Your Energy Field

Here is a simple version for nourishing your energy field with loving, healing energy. Remember, intention is key. Trust and believe the quality of energy you are welcoming is healing. If this feels challenging, save this exercise for a time when it feels more accessible to you. This is an excellent practice to do in nature.

1. Find a peaceful environment to settle into.

2. Take time to deepen your breath and notice how you are feeling.

3. Spend as long as you want mindfully presencing in your body.

4. When you are ready, shift your attention to receiving loving energy from Mother Earth. Imagine energy moving through the soles of your feet, spreading throughout your body, and radiating throughout the farthest reaches of your energy field.

5. When you are ready, invite your spirit guides, healing masters, and guardian ancestors to share their love with you. Make a clear request for every part of you down to the smallest particles to the farthest reaches of your energy fields to be saturated with healing energy.

6. When you feel complete, kindly thank the Earth and your spirit kin for their nurturance.

This simple exercise can leave you feeling energized afterward. For me, I do not do this before bed as I become inspired and invigorated. It can also be calming and grounding. Play with it to see how it best suits your needs.

THREADS THROUGH TIME – ENERGETIC CONNECTIONS

Now that I have spoken about loving versus releasing, I would like to talk about the energetic connections we make with people, places, animals, objects, etc. There is a time when a relationship feels complete, and we are ready to move on. Because we are energetic beings, we form energetic connections with others just as we form physical connections with them. Sometimes these energetic connections effortlessly dissipate when the physical connection ceases. However, other times there is an energetic residue that could benefit from some tending to. I find ritual to be an excellent way to do this. In ritual, we can grieve, appreciate, express unexpressed emotions, celebrate, and bless as we say goodbye. This may feel like the opposite of what we want to do if the relationship was a difficult one. Yet it is an opportunity to reclaim our power and begin reversing disempowering beliefs we may have adopted about ourselves. When and if you are willing to try this practice, it can be empowering and healing.

EXERCISE

Releasing Ritual

In this exercise, I invite you to tap into your inner artist. If reading this stirs up insecurity around artistic expression, press the internal pause button on your inner critic right now. This is not about showcasing a creative piece. It is to invite raw expression as a vehicle for coming to honorable closure with a person, place, etc. that you had a connection with.

Decide what materials you would like to use and gather them. Some options are clay, musical instruments, comfortable clothing for movement, paper and drawing supplies, sewing supplies, collage materials, etc. Carve out plenty of time and space to have an uninterrupted experience. You want to be sure you have time to fully express until you feel complete. Sometimes this is fast and sometimes we tap into a deep reservoir of emotions that requires ample time to express. Depending on the depth of the relationship you are focusing on, you may not want to schedule anything afterward. Consider giving yourself the gift of space to integrate without immediately jumping into another activity. This ritual and the loving-kindness meditation practice (ch.10) are exquisitely complementary in paving the way for a potent experience. I highly recommend beginning (or ending) the ritual with the loving-kindness practice. Read through the exercise first before starting.

1. If you choose, begin with the loving-kindness meditation. Otherwise, take time to get comfortable and presence yourself. Set an intention for this practice.

2. Begin stream-of-consciousness creative expression specific to the emotions evoked when you think of the person. Do your best to get out of your head and let yourself express.

3. Bring forth the full range of emotions felt concerning this person in your expression. "Say" all the things you want to say that you never said (or you felt were not received.) Sing it, dance it, sculpt it, write it, craft it... Leave no words unspoken. Permit yourself to say all the ugly, hurtful, frustrated, painful, rageful things you feel.

4. Take as much time as you need to come to a place where you feel complete.

5. Come back to stillness. If needed, soothe yourself with calming breaths.

6. When you are ready, speak out loud words of letting go and appreciation for all this person, place, etc. has revealed to you about yourself. If this feels uncomfortable, see if you can locate one positive thing you learned from this relationship and focus on gratitude for that. For example: Thank you for loving me when I found it hard to love myself. May you be free from suffering. May I be free from fear of loving. May we all experience joy and love.

7. Notice what sensations you are experiencing and where they are located. For example, you might experience a warm or tingling sensation in your heart center. You might feel a clenching in your gut. Whatever you sense, stay present with it, and breathe.

8. When you feel complete, close the ritual by destroying any physical representation you have. Burn it, let it melt in water, bury it, whatever feels right. You may want to repeat this exercise multiple times related to the same person. Listen and act on what you feel guided to do.

...

Although the concept of energy fields is by no means new, biofield terminology creates an inclusive umbrella for scientific researchers, indigenous healers, energy medicine practitioners, and healthcare providers to explore and converse about these vast networks that are part of and surround every living being. It provides a current framework for indigenous, Eastern, Western, and esoteric philosophies to converge and learn from one another. As we begin to incorporate the existence of energy fields and the communication that occurs within and between them into the way we understand the body, our relationship to healing is radically redefined.

SIX

HEALING OUR ANCESTRAL LINEAGE LINES

Gone were the patterns that held myth, song, ritual, and the poetic imagination as the heartbeat of the people…

…Tending undigested grief of our ancestors not only frees us to live our own lives but also eases ancestral suffering in the other world.

FRANCIS WELLER
The Wild Edge of Sorrow

NOW IS THE TIME

The role of each generation is to be a bridge between the old paradigm and the new consciousness. I believe one of the key evolutionary roles of the generation who are currently parents of young children today is to do intentional healing in our ancestral lineage lines. Of course, it is true of every generation to grow from the last. However, I am referring to a quantum leap in awareness, not the usual next rung on the evolutionary ladder. To best receive the love and wisdom of the luminous souls currently embodying as children, as well as allow the most radical transformation to occur within ourselves, we need to make different choices. We have the chance to take a huge leap in consciousness as a species, to leave behind our caterpillar status and become butterflies. Letting go of outmoded lineage patterns that are alive in our very cells and the unconscious patterns that play out in how we relate to the world, is crucial for gaining this integral perspective.

The opportunity for healing ancestral lines presented in *all* the people I worked with. In my experience, I sense that when a lineage healing occurs, it stretches back to the source regardless of how many generations ago it was. I also believe the impact on future generations, both already born and unborn, is nullified. Peter Levine alluded to this with trauma healing. He said, "the past doesn't matter when we learn how to be present; every moment becomes new and creative. We only have to heal our present symptoms and proceed. A healing moment ripples forward and back, out and about."[1] It is a blessing and a great responsibility for us to take what has been unconsciously repeated and has caused suffering, sometimes over many generations, and lay it to rest. The support and peace I have felt from a client's ancestors when a thread of healing was brought to completion has been astounding. Our ancestors are shining down on each of us with so much love and appreciation for our contribution to collective healing. I believe working with our lineage lines is an essential aspect of lasting change and healing. Healing our lineage lines begins with cultivating a conscious connection with our ancestors. For those of you who do not already have a ritual for connecting with your ancestors, the next exercise is a simple framework for getting started.

EXERCISE

Support from Your Ancestors

There are a lot of ways to cultivate a relationship with your ancestors. Many cultures have maintained practices throughout time that prioritize honoring of their ancestors and asking for their support to gain clarity and wisdom. If you do not already have a practice where you call upon your ancestors for support, this is a great place to start. For this exercise, set an intention to connect with ancestors with whom you had a loving connection. A powerful healing opportunity resides with ancestors we had a challenging relationship with during their lifetime. However, this may take some healing within yourself before you feel ready to meet and receive the guidance/love of these beings. For the sake of initiating connection, keep the practice simple to start.

1. Create an intentional space to get quiet and become present. You may use physical tokens such as setting up an altar space, flowers, crystals, candles, photographs, heirloom objects, etc. Do whatever feels reverent for you.

2. Close your eyes and enter a meditative state. Choose an ancestor to connect with.

3. Connect with the feeling of love you experienced with this person. If you are finding this challenging, choose a specific memory of a time you felt love for this person.

Let yourself return to that moment and remember how you felt as if you were there right now.

4. As you connect with the love, let the memory fade while keeping the feeling of love alive in your heart/body.

5. Now call upon this being to support you with something you want clarity about. For example, perhaps you want to make a life change and don't see what the next step is. Or maybe you simply need to have the courage to take the next step. Ask your ancestor for support and guidance as you traverse this life change.

6. Remain quiet, open, and attentive as you listen for a response. You may get an actual message such as hearing words, a thought, or an image. You may have a feeling of love or warmth wash over you. You may feel a tingling sensation. There are no right or wrong ways to do this. Trust that setting an intention for connection and choosing to be in a receptive state is all that is necessary for your request to be heard. Sometimes it takes some days before a synchronistic event occurs.

7. When you feel complete, close out your experience with an offering of gratitude for your ancestor.

This simple practice connects us with those who came before and initiates a conscious connection with the unseen realms.

CONNECTION WITH SPIRIT

How would it feel to have confidence going through your days that you are supported, and in fact that you have a whole team of guides and masters always available, at your service? Life begins to look very different from this perspective. When it comes time to make big decisions or discover what the next steps are in our lives, we can simply get quiet and ask questions. The responses will come with clarity and ease when our connection with Spirit is activated. We will realize that we are never alone and that we are loved and supported to be the best version of ourselves. Here is Carissa's story.

Carissa's Story – Higher Self Connection

Carissa and I began working together because she wanted to receive spiritual guidance. She had been aware of her sensitivity and connection to Spirit as a child. As she got older, the awareness of this connection faded away. Life happened and she forgot. Skip ahead thirty years to our meeting. She can feel there is so much more for her. She is excited and ready to fulfill the dream of buying a house, being in a loving relationship, and starting a family. By our third session together, Carissa had come to me and said her life is forever changed by the work we are doing together. Her connection with Spirit was blown wide open and she was getting clear communication from her guides about visions of her work in the world, what steps to take next, and opportunities were rapidly being placed before her. She was feeling more connected, inspired, and alive than she could ever remember feeling.

As we continued our work together, Carissa's Spirit guides and Higher Self continued to support her. She began seeing a much bigger contribution that she had to offer in addition to her original vision of home and family. She saw herself as a conservationist and advocate for the Earth. She began weaving together stories and photography, creating beautiful offerings to the community.

During this awakening, Carissa's relationship with herself, her family, and how she interacted with the world drastically shifted. She was able to see where playing the role of caretaker in her family prevented her from seeing herself clearly. She also gained the courage to speak her truth to her family members and co-workers. She didn't feel the need to be the nice one all the time or always "look on the bright side," bypassing her true feelings. By the end of our first cycle of working together, Carissa was a completely different person than when we started. One of the biggest shifts for Carissa was the clarity and confidence she experienced once she felt connected to her Higher Self and her Spirit Guides.

ACTIVATING THE CROWN CHAKRA

The crown chakra, also known as the 7th chakra, resides at the top of the head and is a gateway to our connection with the cosmos. The crown chakra is another area in people that is often congested. I prioritized freeing the crown chakra in my work with others as it can connect them with their guidance and awaken dormant psychic gifts that are an inherent part of their essence. As access to our psychic gifts begins to flow and be sensed again, the world begins to look like a different place. We are now able to make decisions from a place of macrocosmic knowing. We begin to embody the truth of our interconnectedness. This alone is a major shift in consciousness.

When we are born, our crown chakras are wide open. We are between worlds for a little while as we slowly ground into our earthly experience. As we get older and become programmed by societal norms and expectations, often our crown chakra becomes congested by limiting beliefs. We start to dismiss our inner knowing and invalidate our psychic connection as we repeatedly receive the message that what we sense is imaginary. We begin to adopt this version of reality as the truth and our cosmic connection becomes dormant until we do not remember it ever existed. If we do remember, we may have forgotten how to awaken the connection once again. One of the keys to success is being open, rather than dismissive, of whatever form guidance comes in. It takes practice to recognize support when it comes. It takes additional practice to take information in its most raw form, with minimal distortion from the filters of our brains and egos. We can be so desperate to make meaning out of symbols, sensations, etc. that we miss the point of the message altogether. Remember we might not have a logical frame of reference for what we experience in the spiritual domain. Trying to force understanding through a limited perception of understanding is ineffective. It is best to remain curious and open, and allow our frames of reference to expand as fresh perspectives are presented. The next exercise is an invitation to begin awakening your connection with your multi-dimensional family. Try not to take it too seriously. Have fun with it.

EXERCISE

Connecting with Your Higher Self & Spirit Guides

The purpose of this exercise is to create an internal space to receive guidance and to learn to develop trust in the messages of your inner guidance. The first part of the exercise is inspired by Drunvalo Melchizedek's Unity Breath meditation.[2] He received this meditation in a vision from Sri Yukteswar of the Kriya Yoga lineage.

1. Find a comfortable seated position, inside or outside.

2. Close your eyes and begin to relax, finding a gentle rhythm to your breathing.

3. Connect in your heart space. Spend at least a few breaths here arriving and quieting the mind.

4. Now shift your attention to the appreciation and awe you have for all life that exists beyond the Earth.

5. With your intention, send love and appreciation from your heart, through the top of your head, into the vast cosmos.

6. Now *receive* the love from the cosmos back into your heart through your crown chakra. Continue to cycle this exchange of energy between your heart and the cosmos.

7. You may stop here and practice this first part of the exercise to bring awareness and awakening to the crown chakra.

8. As you are ready, call upon your guides and higher self, using your words, either out loud or in your head. For example, I say, "I cast a golden sphere of light around me that allows only energies coming in highest service to my highest healing and the highest healing for all. I call forth my higher self and my guides to support me now." Create an invocation that resonates for you. You may also simply wait to receive any guidance that comes forth.

9. Now you can either ask a question you are seeking support around or ask your guides if they have a message for you that would be helpful for you to know now. Have patience and receptivity as you sense any information that comes. Again, it may be in the form of a feeling, a sound, an image, a thought, or a sensation. Whatever the form, acknowledge it as real, not your imagination. As you develop this relationship with your unseen guardians, you may begin to recognize patterns of communication and decipher what they mean for you.

10. End your practice with appreciation for your guides and know that they are always there loving you, supporting you, and presenting opportunities for your growth.

IMPRINTS THROUGH TIME

Our heritage has a much greater impact on us than we are aware of. It is not a mystery that genetics influence our physical makeup. In addition to physical attributes, our DNA is imprinted *energetically* through time. In the emerging field of epigenetics, scientists have recently validated what healers have been aware of and addressing through the ages. Our behaviors and environment have an undeniable impact on the expression of our DNA, therefore affecting our physical, emotional, and spiritual health.

The energetic influences of our lineage lines must be addressed to achieve lasting personal healing and generational transformation. Which genes get activated is influenced by our lineage impressions. We do not need to carry the weight of the past on the shoulders of our present or into the future. However, to do this we need to become aware of these influential patterns and take them as seriously as we would physical symptoms. In Grace's story, she experienced intense physical symptoms during pregnancy that I believe was her body and the incoming soul's way of communicating to her an opportunity to heal a lineage imprint.

Grace's Story – Prenatal Illness & Breech Presentation

Grace first came to me two months before her baby was due. It was her first pregnancy and she had been experiencing daily vomiting and exhaustion since the first few weeks of the pregnancy. On most days she was unable to eat much food without throwing it back up and was therefore concerned about the nourishment she and the baby were receiving. In general, Grace was a highly fit, healthy young woman. She had an excellent diet, was in a loving relationship, and was very happy with the work she was doing in the world. There were no obvious (or conventional) reasons why she would be feeling this ill past the common first-trimester symptoms. I knew from the first moment Grace and I talked there was an ancestral lineage connection contributing to her illness.

We did one session with Grace that focused on lineage connections as the possible root of her nausea. She had connections on both her maternal and paternal sides that presented. I sensed the connection with her paternal grandmother was the main contributing factor influencing the vomiting. However, there was also a connection with her maternal grandfather in her heart chakra. This was causing an emotional barrier to fully opening herself to the baby. After this one session of working with these lineage ties, Grace felt completely different. The baby was moving significantly more than she had felt her before. The vomiting ceased and she was able to enjoy her pregnancy for the first time. She remained energized and felt well for the remainder of her pregnancy.

During this first session, I became aware of two more sessions that could provide important emotional support before Grace gave birth. There were more lineage pieces she was ready to shed. Six weeks after our first session, Grace came in for another. Again, I could sense lineage pieces on both sides of Grace's family. Fear was the theme of this session. There was a fear thread present from both paternal lines and a maternal line. The fear was specifically related to giving birth. We addressed this emotional energy and focused healing energy on her and the baby.

Grace came to the third session at 38 weeks having just discovered the night before that the baby turned breech. She was hoping for support in either shifting the baby's position or finding peace that this is how the baby would enter the world. During the first part of the session, we completed working with the lineage fear on her maternal side. I sensed that there was a breech birth farther back in this lineage. I also sensed that Grace's baby did not need to be born breech as a way for the lineage line to receive deeper healing.

During the second part of our session, I asked Grace to get down on her hands and knees. I joined her and became acutely aware of the baby's experience. We began with small movements and stretches. Eventually, the rocking and twisting of my body intensified. While I was energetically connected with the baby,

Grace was feeling the movements of the baby within her womb mirroring the movements I was making. My body movements went from rocking to a swift, smooth, spiral motion, landing the baby in the desired head-down position. It felt like I was guiding the baby on the path to head-down. That day, the baby shifted a quarter turn toward head-down.

Over the next few days, I did remote sessions with Grace and her baby. Each time she could feel the baby responding to my movements. Each time, the baby turned a little more. In the meantime, Grace was trying all the recommended ideas from her midwives with no luck. Finally, four days after her last in-person session, and with the support of some physical manipulation, the baby moved into the head-down position. A few days later, Grace gave birth to a healthy baby girl, naturally at home, in a head-down position.

The healing opportunity for Grace during this pregnancy was to work with lineage fears that presented before her daughter's birth. Because of Grace's willingness to explore lineage healing, her daughter was born more fully embodying a legacy of love.

Grace's story was a quick healing that occurred in a few sessions with few side effects. Although she was unwell for many months as she navigated what was really at the root of her discomfort, once the healing occurred, Grace and her baby were free from the weight of ancestral fear (and frequent vomiting.) This is not how it always goes. Sometimes things appear worse before they get better. It is not unusual to experience flare-ups during a deep release and healing process. This is an important thing to be aware of, as sometimes *where* the flare-up occurs is seemingly unrelated. This next story is a personal experience where inflammation occurred in a predictable place, however, it could easily have been misconstrued as something unrelated to the healing work I had been doing.

My Story – Cervix Inflammation, Shame, & Sexuality

A few years ago, I went to have an annual pap smear checkup. It came back as abnormal and the doctor recommended I receive a colposcopy (a procedure to more closely examine my cervix) for further analysis. During the weeks before, I had begun a deep lineage healing that included all four strands of my ancestral lines. I was specifically addressing the emotion of shame as related to sexuality. I discovered a large concentration of emotional energy housed in my cervix. I was deep in this process of working with shame when I went to get the pap smear. It was no surprise to me that the doctor discovered inflammation on my cervix. I followed her recommendation to get a colposcopy as a precaution. However, I waited three weeks before I scheduled it, as I received clear guidance that I was still in the process of releasing and healing, and my body needed time for the inflammation to subside. Three weeks later, I went to get the procedure. She found small traces of inflammation still there but said, "I have nothing to worry about. All is well." A year later when I went to receive my annual follow-up exam, everything came back perfectly clear.

Having the awareness that lineage imbalances significantly impact us, as well as the commitment to address them, is a vital part of experiencing healing and evolution both as an individual and as a species. Lineage patterns have a profound impact on us whether we are conscious of the pattern or not. We can let them remain unconscious or welcome the awareness that our lineage is alive in us, and we have the power to discard patterns that are not aligned with our values. When we choose the latter, it enables us to transform our lives and those of the future generations.

EXERCISE

Make a New Choice

When there is clarity gained about a lineage pattern, the primary way to etch a new path moving forward is by making new choices. Having support (such as a practitioner of lineage healing or a therapist) can help provide clarity and build momentum. Regardless, the most influential aspect is to consistently choose new behaviors that reflect what you truly desire. It's one thing to recognize a lineage pattern and another to make a different choice that is not reactionary but a new construct altogether.

1. Once you are clear on what the lineage pattern is, write down both the pattern and the version of yourself that you are excited to embrace that is not influenced by this pattern.

2. Next, create an action list that this new version of you would do. For example, let's say you identified a communication pattern of shutting down when you felt vulnerable. You linked this to a lineage pattern. It was a behavior you remember your mom doing and your grandmother before her. For your whole life, you too have been unconsciously reenacting this generational response. Now, let's say you are in an interaction and you sense the shutdown is about to happen. Instead of continuing on autopilot, you do a pattern interrupt. You pause, take 10 deep breaths before continuing to interact, and then meet the conversation with receptivity. If you

need more time or space, repeat the 10 breaths. The pausing and taking 10 deep breaths can now go on your list of action steps.

3. Put into practice the actions on your list. Which ones are effective? Which ones come more easily? Do you need to make alterations for the action to become more effective? Continue to add to and refine the list as needed.

Ultimately, you do not need more than one action if it is effective, and you use it. Lineage patterns have momentum. An effective way to change the direction of your ship and build momentum in this new direction is to choose actions that are simple and clear. The more you practice the new actions, the more natural they will become. Eventually, you will not need to think about it as it becomes fully integrated into the new version of you.

SEVEN

EMBODYING OUR SEXUAL POWER

Azeza, our son, was born in the Atlantic Ocean. The night was dark and clear as the crystalline ocean washed warm waves over our shoulders. Orion, the protector of the sky, kept watch over our timeless moment. I felt calm in the infinite vastness of the ocean. Held by the water, I felt the oneness of life. We all experienced this union in the absolute silence between contractions, in the total surrender that is the moment of emergence. A manta ray circled our birthing triangle, assisting us in creating a sacred space in the water. The perfection of this moment was total magic. Azeza arrived at 6:24 AM as the sun lit a soft glow on the horizon. We crossed the threshold of the sea and land as reverent parents.

A RETURN TO THE SACRED

The above excerpt is from a story that I co-wrote with my ex-husband in 2009 describing the pregnancy and birth of our first child. It was a miraculous gestation period guided by deep, intuitive listening that culminated in birthing him in the warm waters of the Atlantic Ocean just north of Miami, Florida. My pregnancy was the first time I can remember feeling the deep wisdom that lies within my womb.

As a girl, I grew up demoralized by the way I witnessed men, specifically my father, treating women. Before long, I was objectified and terrified by the disempowering dynamic between men and women. I learned to believe the only way to obtain the love of a man was to submit my body to whatever sexual pleasure he wanted. I also learned to dissociate from my body during any sexual contact. This began with my 8-year-old self getting a forceful, unwanted kiss from a classmate while pressed up against a tree in the woods. I had a rough entry into this world of being a girl. Sadly, my story is not uncommon in today's longstanding patriarchal culture.

Healing my relationship with my sexuality has been the most painstaking task I have encountered. It has taken me decades to unravel all the unconscious beliefs laden with shame I absorbed from my earliest experiences. It has taken me years to come home to myself and inhabit the body that seemed to threaten the tenderest parts of me. It has required immense patience to let my vulnerability emerge in its own timing.

My embodiment process has been a precious journey of deep healing for me, my past lineage, and now my children. The birth of my son was one of the majestic fruits of my labor. It was a powerful rite of passage not only from maiden to mother, but also in trusting my body, my intuition, and my spiritual guidance. It was single handedly the most powerful, transformational experience of my life because I now *knew* the true power of being a woman. My pregnancy and his birth inspired me to continue my exploration of this sacred space and to access the cosmic connection that resides in the womb.

(To clarify, my journey was a culmination of years of sexual, emotional, and spiritual healing that happened to coalesce in an empowering, life-altering birthing experience. Whether a person chooses to have a child or not has no bearing on the journey they can take in embodying their sexual power.)

WOMB WISDOM

Soon after becoming pregnant, I felt the awakening of a cellular memory that our sexual energy is a superhighway connector to the multi-dimensions and the divine. I could feel the magnitude of potentiality in having a conscious connection with our sexual energy to communicate with Spirit. It was beyond the act of physical pleasure and could equally be explored with a partner or alone. I realized that I had a deep-seated fear of the power of my sexual energy and specifically of my feminine sexual energy. Something cracked open inside of me during the journey of labor. It became clear to me that I needed to remember the full power of the womb if I was going to embody my fullest potential in this lifetime.

After giving birth, I was guided to various teachers and texts to assist me on my journey of unlocking this potential within. I fervently studied and practiced supportive exercises to awaken my 2nd chakra energy. The work of Tami Lynn Kent and her book, *Wild Feminine*, opened a door to a whole other universe.[1] I soaked in her words and worked with the exercises in her book. Inspired by my deepening womb connection, I began facilitating groups of women to reconnect with their wombs. During our time together, we traversed individual and collective trauma held in the womb space. The healing that happened for all of us was profound.

One of the main healings that occurred in the group was the need for a conscious, more consistent spiritual connection with Mother Earth. All the women in the group were the type who spent a lot of time in nature and had a reverence for the Earth. They already believed the Earth to be a conscious being who is co-creating with us on our earth journey. However, the type of connection I am referring to went deeper than this fundamental understanding. It was a connection to unconditional love. It was a knowing that Mother Earth could be relied upon for support to transmute the anger, grief, and fear we felt. She had an unlimited capacity to hold us in anything we were experiencing.

This was the first time many of the women had received this level of love and support. Cultivating a connection with the Earth enabled us to feel the pain that was stored in our womb spaces. The womb is a storehouse for grief: our grief, our family's grief, and our collective grief as well. Together, we accessed shame, fear, and unworthiness while being held by one another and Mother Earth as emotional energy released from the sanctuary of the womb. This made way for hope, inspiration, and the possibility for the voice of the womb to be heard.

A constant dynamic of the healing journey is the ebb and flow of activation, integration, restoration, and inspiration. During these groups, we integrated individual and collective trauma related to being a woman. As this occurred, space was made for new, empowered choices that encouraged us to stand more fully in our feminine power and let our voices be heard. Every woman who participated in the journey was transformed. They left with a fresh understanding of the power of the womb and how to nurture and express this power.

EXERCISE

Energetic Womb Cleansing

This exercise is a wonderful practice to provide self-care and ongoing maintenance of your womb space. Read through the exercise first and then begin.

Energetic womb cleansing is equally powerful for those who have had hysterectomies. At the time of writing this book, I had not received feedback from any trans-woman using this practice. I therefore do not know what the experience might be like. However, I do imagine that if you feel a connection to a womb space in your body, this practice would be powerful and beneficial.

1. Find a comfortable sitting position, either on the floor or in a chair. Close your eyes and connect with your breath.

2. Begin to gently rock your pelvis - back and forth, side to side, allowing a conscious connection with your womb space to begin happening.

3. Now find stillness and take five even breaths into your heart space.

4. Visualize a ball of light in your heart. Notice the qualities the ball has – color, texture, etc. When you are ready, use your intention to move this ball of light down the center of your body into your womb space.

5. Once inside, shine this light around to all sides of your womb space. Leave no corner untouched. If you sense anything in your womb that feels shadowy or uncomfortable, spend some extra time there. Perhaps there is something that wants to be communicated to you about this area? Explore and ask. Remember to be gentle and loving. Be alert for any pushiness slipping in and soften it with spaciousness and your breath.

6. You can take the time to cleanse all areas of your womb in any way you are inspired to. For example, you can imagine yourself using a duster or broom, misting with your favorite essential oils, or perhaps lighting a fire in the center and discarding any unwanted findings into the fire. The options are infinite. Whatever inspires you is perfect.

7. When you feel satisfied with a general "house cleaning" of your womb, you can summon a sacred object to place in your womb space. Again, be creative and put something there that feels empowering. This is a part of reclaiming your womb as a sacred space.

8. Lastly, take time to nourish your womb with gratitude and appreciation for the marvelous power it has to create.

FINDING OUR VOICE - PRACTICING CONSENT

It is never too early (or too late) to begin practicing consent. As children, we receive many messages that we do not have authority over what happens to our bodies. Perhaps we are pushed into giving a family member a hug or our sibling holds us down, not respecting our no. As a mother of two who values teaching consent to my son and daughter, I have seen many challenges arise in the microcosm of our family related to consent. I often ask myself, "what are my kids learning about consent and how will they take the experiences they learn at home into the world?" One thing to keep in mind is consent is woven into the fabric of every human-to-human interaction. It is applicable beyond sexual association. The best rule of thumb is there is never too much asking for consent.

Consent creates safety within to communicate our vulnerabilities and swaddle our fears that inadvertently arise when we authentically express ourselves. Consent is a key missing element in how we habitually treat one another. This has led to a society rampant with coercion, manipulation, domination, and influencing as acceptable norms. These actions can be extremely subtle and completely unconscious, yet they are felt as overtly as a door being slammed in our faces. When confronted by someone who plows over our voice, needs, and desires, we are left feeling silenced, disempowered, and oftentimes, violated. The power dynamic of not asking for consent creates unbearable suffering in our world. It is the energy that starts wars, rapes, colonizes, destroys, pollutes, bullies, patronizes, and brutalizes. Practicing consent in our daily lives has the potential to initiate a ripple effect that is profound within our intimate relationships, families, and communities. It is an act of saying I matter, and you matter too.

> Practicing consent in our daily lives has the potential to initiate a ripple effect that is profound within our intimate relationships, families, and communities. It is an act of saying I matter, and you matter too.

In addition to asking for consent, learning to celebrate a person's response, whether it is a yes or no, is validating, empowering, and can be profoundly healing. One of my mentors, Marla Mattenson,[2] does an exceptional job emphasizing the importance of consistent consent and celebrating all responses. In the world we live in, it can take courage to articulate a no. Many of us have our lives centered around saying yes to the things we think we *should* do, rather than doing what truly inspires us. For a variety of reasons, we fear setting a boundary, saying no, and claiming what we truly desire. This behavior leads to a whole host of imbalances in all areas of our lives.

LIFESTYLE TIP

Just Ask

There are two aspects to begin practicing consent: listening and asking.

- Notice the times during your day you do not ask for consent. What are the circumstances? Who is it with?

- Notice the times during the day when you witness others not asking for consent. How did the other person respond?

- Choose one person for a whole day whom you will ask for consent before doing anything with/for them. If you have a child(ren), perhaps you could practice with them. Notice how they respond? Is it different than you are accustomed to?

- Celebrate them when they respond no! Celebrate them when they respond yes! Do not question them or try to change their mind if the answer is different than you hoped for. Do not ask a question if you are not open to receiving a no.

- Make a request from someone you trust for them to ask you for consent before making assumptions, interrupting, or taking over.

CREATING SAFETY WITHIN

Consent is a crucial component of creating safety within. In addition, becoming skilled at tending to our inner selves has a significant impact on creating safety within. As we do this, we come to trust ourselves to set healthy boundaries and listen to the needs of our vulnerable aspects. It is the marriage of asking for consent from our inner selves and nurturing them with love and boundary setting that creates and upholds safety. Once we know how to keep ourselves safe, we no longer search outside of ourselves in the form of a partner, parent, or other for safety. As this occurs, our capacity to open to receiving immensely increases.

OPENING TO RECEIVING

Many of us have surrounded our hearts with protective barriers from heartbreaks and traumas that occurred as children. At the time, this was an excellent strategy for coping with emotions that were overwhelming for us to process. However, for most of us, these strategic, behavioral patterns are no longer necessary and frequently cause disruption and inner turmoil. In addition, they limit our capacity to receive. After all, a well-built fortress is intended to keep *everything* out. This includes love, health, pleasure, wealth, grief, joy, etc. It also traps everything in, constricting the flow of the vast array of emotional experiences. This leaves us living a life of mediocracy and increases the likelihood of stagnation of emotional energy.

The arena of sex and sexuality is saturated with copious amounts of shunning and shaming. Many repress their desires for fear of being judged or being "too much." As children, we may have been shamed for touching ourselves or for our sexual curiosity. Some cultures have failed at normalizing sexual desire and activity. This burdens adults with a buildup of sexual energy that is sometimes released in disempowered and harmful ways.

Frequently, women I have worked with do not know what it is they desire sexually or what brings them sensual pleasure. Many have never touched their bodies in a sensual way; just the thought of self-pleasuring can initiate a cascade of intense physiological responses based on the fear of being wrong or shamed. Getting in touch with what we desire can require patience and tenderness.

There is a myriad of beliefs all genders have adopted that lead to resisting pleasure, love, and joy. The most insidious may be not believing we are worthy of it. This leads us back to the shame conversation in chapter 2. Embodying our sexual power will likely include navigating inner dialogues with parts of ourselves harboring shame.

Below is an exercise that invites an exploration of our sensual side. It does not have to lead to a sexual experience, although it could. Remember to honor your pacing. If you begin to feel uncomfortable sensations (physical or emotional), slow down or stop. Perhaps take time with any inner selves emerging and see what your body is communicating to you. Maybe place your hand on your heart and do a grounding exercise to help you stay present and feel safe. The intention of this practice is to have it feel good. Only do what brings you a sense of curiosity and pleasure.

EXERCISE

Non-Gender Specific Self-Pleasure Practice

Getting to know your body is an important part of discovering what brings you pleasure. Many of us were not encouraged to explore our bodies. Some of us explored them privately fearing the shame of being caught. Some had experiences so young they have no memory of not feeling betrayed by their body. Wherever you land on the spectrum of sensual exploration, let this practice be a chance to discover something new about yourself.

This practice is intended to be done alone. It is to become better acquainted with your sensual side. Even if you feel confident in this area, give it a try. You may be pleasantly surprised by what you discover. Play and have fun.

1. Create a space where you have privacy and will feel safe doing whatever spontaneously arises.

2. Gather any objects you are curious to explore with. Keep in mind this is not necessarily a sexual exploration, but rather a sensual one (that may lead to a sexual one.) Some ideas for objects are foods that bring you pleasure, materials/objects with a texture you enjoy, music that excites you, etc.

3. Take a few moments grounding and set an intention for the practice. If it is helpful, check in with any inner selves that may be activated by this practice. Reassure them they are safe, and you will take care of them.

4. Do a body scan. Are there any places that feel tense/
    uncomfortable? If so, spend some time gently breathing
    into these places. If the tension does not dissipate, be sure
    to remain attentive to the sensation as you continue. If
    it increases in intensity, stop, and sense what would best
    serve your needs.

5. When (and if) you are ready, begin to explore with your
    senses. Maybe you want to play with smell as you smell
    a scent that brings you pleasure. Maybe you want to feel
    what different objects feel like as you gently (or roughly)
    move them against your bare skin. Perhaps you want to
    take a bite of fruit and let the juice run down your chin
    and neck. Whatever you explore, pay close attention to
    your senses. Really hone in on what you are feeling. For
    example, do you like the way the juice feels or is the
    stickiness gross to you? Play and discover what brings
    you pleasure.

6. If you feel inclined, use your hands to caress different parts
    of your body. Where are your erogenous zones today?
    Explore how different pressures feel in different places.

7. If at any point you feel yourself slipping away and
    becoming less present, stop. Breathe. Listen. What do
    you need right now to stay present in your felt senses?
    If you continue, go slowly, and notice the edge of when
    you begin to disconnect. This is useful information.
    Awareness is the starting point of healing.

8. You may feel sexual energy building as you explore.
    You can choose to have an orgasm if you want,

however, I encourage you to take time to explore the subtler sensations before shifting gears. Some of us habitually kick into an automated version of sex that does not take into consideration what pleases us. Slow down and really lavish yourself with sensations that are erotic and arousing.

There are no wrong ways to do this exercise. It is about discovery, curiosity, and liberation. Depending on your past experiences, this could bring up strong emotions for you. Please go slow and take care of yourself. If any emotions arise that feel too overwhelming to navigate, ask for support from a trusted friend or professional guide.

TAKING OUR POWER BACK

Being in touch with what we desire is being connected with our instincts and our animal nature. We have long been shamed out of embodying our animal nature, yet it is a fundamental part of what makes us human. Women especially have been persecuted for expressing their sexual, sensual, and powerful nature. It has instilled fear in many of us. Knowing what we desire, sexually and otherwise, is essential for taking our power back. Deep down, we know exactly what we desire. Our instincts reside underneath all the stories, beliefs, programs, and fears. As we peel back the layers of the fortress, we begin to sense a stirring.

For the benefit of all humankind, as well as our emotional and physical well-being, rejecting good girl status and getting in touch with our wild side is pivotal.

Kasia Urbaniak developed a gorgeous body of work that educates women about "good girl conditioning" and how to break free[3]. Urbaniak stated some qualities of the good girl as selfless, accommodating, appropriate, upbeat, low-maintenance, harmonizing, never out-shining others, maintaining the status quo, conflict avoidant, and an expert at making do. She continued by breaking down the origin of good girl conditioning (which was a literal manual teaching girls how to be marriable.) This programming leaves all genders at a disadvantage because we fear expressing the fullness of who we are. Deprogramming from "good girl conditioning" is an arduous, inspiring, and meaningful task that takes courage. For the benefit of all humankind, as well as our emotional and physical well-being, rejecting good girl status and getting in touch with our wild side is pivotal. This is true for all genders.

LIFESTYLE TIP

Exploring Your Wild Side

Exploring your wild side is fueled by one thing: curiosity. It is incredibly liberating and can be a little bit terrifying. Being willing to let your wild side be witnessed (even by yourself) takes courage. We have all been shamed into taming our instinctual nature. Ask yourself these questions to begin exploring your wild side.

- What do you need to feel safe letting out a primal yell?

- Are you afraid to let the sound of your pleasure be fully expressed during sex?

- Is there any environment where you feel able to fully let loose? For example, if you are grieving can you allow yourself to wail with your whole being?

- Can you set the judgmental part of yourself aside that fears what others might think and let yourself move your body/dance with wild abandon?

We can uncage ourselves. Beginning to understand our limitations around letting our wild sides free will indicate what the next step is towards letting our animal nature have its rightful spot at the dining table.

SEXUAL ENERGY & WELLNESS

Embodying our sexual power has a profound influence on our wellness. There are overt ways this is true such as having satisfying sexual relationships that foster pleasure rather than harm and establishing a loving relationship with our bodies. Additionally, there are many less obvious ways embodying our sexual power impacts our wellness.

One can imagine the immense power our sexual energy has by contemplating the mere fact that it is with this magnificent force that human vessels are created. When creations such as children are made from sexual energy that is even mildly flowing, imagine the opposite effect that can occur when it is stifled. Furthermore, imagine the magnitude of possibility when our sexual energy flows with empowered fluidity and focused direction.

The potential to harness our sexual energy to nourish and rejuvenate our bodies is astonishing. It can be redirected for healing the body and fueling creative pursuits with its life-giving capacity. In addition, sexual energy can be cultivated to have profound spiritual experiences. The Taoist lineage has shared with the world many practices on working with sexual energy. Mantak and Maneewan Chia have books detailing ancient practices of cultivating sexual energy[4,5]. These practices begin with solo cultivation.

The relationship is in knowing thyself first. Learning how to circulate sexual energy throughout the body is a powerful practice for supercharging the physical body and energy fields.

> The potential to harness our sexual energy to nourish and rejuvenate our bodies is astonishing. It can be redirected for healing the body and fueling creative pursuits with its life-giving capacity.

We live in a world fraught with sexual trauma including the silencing of sexual expression by shaming. When our traumatic sexual experiences are left unintegrated, the emotional, energetic, and physical ripples can be devastating to our vitality and overall health. These effects go beyond our sexual interactions. They can leave us dissociated from our bodies, out of touch with our needs and desires, feeling unworthy of love, and afraid of physical touch. Throughout the years I have seen many clients who experienced sexual trauma that had chronic conditions including being overweight, ovarian cancer, and severe anxiety and depression. Unlocking the potential of our sexual power is not only a great benefit for maximizing our health, it is a necessity.

EIGHT

EMPOWERMENT TOOLS AND STRATEGIES

As we say a courageous yes to growth, we need to continue to take new action steps that support the changes we are inspired to embody. Evolution is not a one-time deal. It is an infinite spiral with opportunities for growth being revealed all the time. Making changes can be terrifying and exciting. Having tools and strategies for when fear arises will facilitate more grace in the transitions.

There are an infinite number of tools and strategies. In this book thus far, there are many valuable exercises to put in your self-care toolkit. Some additional strategies I consistently use are meditation, visualization, updating my environment, clear communication, and boundary setting.

MEDITATION

We must make time to listen. Meditation allows us to tune into our bodies and sense what is being communicated. Sometimes the feelings are subtle and if we do not still ourselves and listen, we will not hear the valuable messages being shared. We have been trained to push through our days and ignore how we are feeling. Sometimes this behavior is even praised, as we are encouraged to push through the pain. Our bodies always tell us when we are out of alignment. At first, it begins as a whisper. The whispers get louder and louder until our bodies are screaming at us in pain. If we discipline ourselves to consistently listen, many imbalances can be caught in the early stages never resulting in physical symptoms. If we allow ourselves to feel emotions as they arise and listen to the roots of physical pain, we can let energy move through us. Not repressing the flow of energy can help us avoid problems later. Having a meditation practice is an excellent way to listen to ourselves.

Meditation also allows us to become quiet enough to connect with our spirit guides and higher selves. Again, their messages frequently have a subtle expression, so it is important to cultivate deep listening skills. Having a conscious connection with our multi-dimensional allies is an invaluable tool for navigating life and staying in alignment with our values, gifts, and purpose.

A meditation practice can look a variety of ways. It can be walking, sitting, or lying down. It can be with our eyes open or closed. We can use our breath as a focal point, or not. The main point is to find a way of meditating that is easy to commit to doing. Some people believe they cannot meditate, and that it does not work for them. One of the reasons this belief exists is the misleading idea that the mind must be empty of all thoughts. This is very difficult to do. Meditation does not require our mind to be completely quiet, rather it requires a redirection of our attention when distracting thoughts come up. Choosing something to return your focus to is helpful. Some examples are the breath, the heart, a peaceful place, gratitude for a person/place, or a candle. There are no right or wrong ways to do this, relax and let it be easy. You may even need to call it something different than meditation to invite yourself to let go of any expectations you are placing upon yourself and the experience. Simply get quiet and gently breathe.

VISUALIZATION

While meditation is for listening, visualization is for initiating action. How we visualize things has a tremendous impact on what comes to pass. This includes things we want and do not want to happen. Our brain does not discern between imaginary scenarios we visualize and scenarios that are "real." We can use this to our advantage. When we can visualize the outcomes we desire and do this repeatedly, the chances of successful manifestation increase. Remember, every physical manifestation begins as a thought. The more we focus our mind's eye on exactly what we desire and the more palpably we can feel our manifested results with our full senses, the faster they will come into physical form. Think of visualization as a navigational compass directing us to our destination points. As we are sailing, we need to continually adjust and monitor the bearings to account for variables. Similarly, visualizing with consistency while keeping our attention focused on what we want and refining our goals as we gain more clarity about what we desire will lead us to our destination points. Our ship is sailing one way or the other. Would you rather be at the helm navigating towards the point of your destination? Or would you rather abandon the helm and hope that you do not shipwreck into the rocks? Visualization is a key tool for taking us where we want to be. This is true for all aspects of our lives be it health, relationships, work, or lifestyle goals. The next exercise is an opportunity to play with what inspires you and to begin embodying these desires.

EXERCISE

Imagining the Life You Desire

Being able to clearly visualize the life you desire and then embody it, with emotion, as if it is real now, is a huge part of actualizing the life you desire. This is not new news. You will read it in just about any book sharing how to manifest and create something you want. However, reading about something and putting it into practice are two very different things. Here is a simple visualization exercise to get your focus fine-tuned, your intention set, and momentum building toward the life you desire.

1. If you are not clear on what you want to create in your life, the first step is to spend time asking yourself questions and dreaming up the best-case scenario you can imagine for the different areas of your life. You can meditate, journal, do vision boards, or watch/read inspiring stories to spark your inspiration. It is well worth spending time to get clear on what you want. Clarity is crucial for creating it. The more details you have the better. If you do not have a visual, but you are clear on the *feeling* of what you want, that's great. Stay focused on the feeling. It is important to focus only on what you are clear about. For example, if you know you want a new house that has two floors and a lot of light, focus on that and how you feel in this new home. More clarity will come the more you ponder the question and the more you do this exercise. Let your vision flush out naturally and authentically. Use feelings of expansion, love, excitement,

and inspiration as guiding lights indicating you are on the right track to something aligned and meaningful.

2. Once you are clear, choose a time and a space where you can commit to doing this practice in a focused way every day. Adding it to a meditation practice is fantastic, as you already will be centered with your attention turned inward.

3. Once you are in a connected and receptive state, begin to visualize yourself in the life you desire as if it is your life now. For example, if you want a different house, go through a day in the life of your new house with as many details as possible. Most importantly how do you feel doing the thing you desire?

   Examples of questions to ask yourself are:

   - What clothes am I wearing to feel amazing?
   - How is my house decorated?
   - What food am I eating?
   - What activities am I doing throughout the day to feel most vital?
   - How do I interact with my partner, my family?
   - What kind of friend am I?
   - What does my bank account look like when I view it?
   - How am I being of service to the world?
   - What brings me joy?
   - What brings me pleasure?
   - What does my thriving sex life look like?

4. As you are flushing out your vision, add the other senses to your experience. What does it sound like in your

environment? How do your clothes feel against your skin? What does pleasure taste like? What does your skin warming in the sun smell like? Use your senses to make the experience even more vivid.

5. As you are arriving more fully into this scenario you have created, allow yourself to have an emotional experience of what it feels like to live in this version of your life. This is a crucial part of manifesting. Let joy, pleasure, ecstasy, inspiration, gratitude, love, etc. swell inside of your being.

6. Continue to practice this visualization as often as possible. You can begin to incorporate the essence of your vision into moments throughout your day. You can look at yourself in the mirror as the person who already lives that life. You can begin choosing items in your environment that match the essence of your vision. For example, you can buy new articles of clothes, bedding, or different foods. You can begin relating differently to others now as the new you.

There are always actions you can take toward the life circumstances you desire that will build momentum and bring you closer to your goal. Remember that how you feel in your new life is always more important than the items in it. Focusing on the felt sense and pleasurable emotions is what brings your dreams more quickly into form.

TAKING ACTION

There are two parts to making a change: doing internal work to gain increased awareness and taking action based on this new awareness. We could spend the rest of our lives receiving healing work or reading personal development books and still never see the changes we desire. Why? Because someone else cannot fix us. To have true and lasting change we must act by making new choices.

Action plans look differently for each of us. Ideally, they are inspired by our gifts and life purpose combined with external circumstances that excite us and bring us joy. Though an action plan is logistical, it does not mean it has to be logical. Oftentimes the steps of our plan come from an intuitive knowing and they may not make sense to our minds at all. Sometimes taking action is terrifying because it requires vulnerability. Taking action means interacting with the world. This means people may judge us. We will have failures. We will expose ourselves to be of service. Some people will feel uncomfortable with our choices. We may challenge the status quo. We will make mistakes. Given the number of traumatizing experiences most of us have had, exposing our dreams to others can be downright debilitating. This is where the skill of knowing how to tend to our inner selves is crucial.

Taking action is a courageous act of self-love. It is standing up loud and proud in our worthiness. It is taking the role of leader, a leader of love. The type of actions we are taking are life-affirming and will not intentionally harm another or ourselves. The tasks in our plan regardless of how big or small are symbolic of something much greater. They represent the belief in ourselves that we have a worthy contribution to make during our lifetime. What actions can you take right now, that you have been hesitating about, that you know will bring you closer to your goal?

MAKING CHANGES IN OUR ENVIRONMENT

Making changes in our environment that embody the person we want to become is an important aspect of creating lasting change in our lives. This can be intimidating depending on the magnitude of the change being made *and* it is an absolute necessity to consistently make choices that are an energetic match to the new frequency we are aspiring to embody.

For example, you may have a bed that you think is uncomfortable. It has old hand-me-down sheets on it and a comforter you bought at the thrift store 10 years earlier. You are very aware that you awake most days feeling a little achy in your body because you have a worn-out mattress. When you walk into your bedroom you do not feel a sense of excitement and joy about the beautiful, comfortable bed you have. Instead, it either goes unnoticed or you even dread sleeping in it another night. Get rid of that bed! Take the time to find a mattress, bedding, and pillows that are both aesthetically pleasing and where you feel like royalty sleeping in it. You can apply this example to any number of things such as outmoded relationships, jobs, material items, attitudes, locations, communication patterns, etc.

There are an infinite number of changes we can make to our environment that embrace the person we are becoming. Do not underestimate the ripple effect these changes can have regardless of how large or small they seem. When we claim our self-worth by surrounding ourselves with people, places, and things we love and feel inspired by, our dreams begin to become our reality.

LIFESTYLE TIP

Make One Change Daily

- Make at least one change to your environment each day to support being the person you want to become.

- Invite more uplifting activities, relationships, and places into your day-to-day.

- Simultaneously, release activities, relationships, objects, etc. that are draining you.

- Remember to do a balanced amount of letting go of things and welcoming in the new.

Continue to have a practice like this throughout your life. You are changing and growing all the time and therefore want to use your environment to support and reflect the newest version of yourself.

CLEAR COMMUNICATION

It is essential to express what we need. If we do not express what we need, we attract relationships and situations where either we put others' needs before our own and/or others feel responsible to guess what we need. This leads to disempowerment and imbalance for all parties. We cannot have the loving, fulfilled relationships we desire without taking this very important action of empowered, clear communication seriously. Once we express our desires, the other person may or may not be able to support these requests. Ideally, we will be in relationships where there is at least a willingness to hear our requests and be as supportive as possible. However, whether other people show up in a supportive role or not, ultimately is irrelevant. When we express our needs clearly and then take action to support these desires getting met, we are honoring ourselves. This is what is most important.

Clear communication is also a crucial aspect of taking responsibility in relationships. When we do not express our needs clearly, it is easy to project resentment, anger, and frustration on others for our needs not being met. Underlying this, deep grief builds from not expressing ourselves. Some of us have no idea what we even want. It then becomes difficult to communicate our needs to others since we do not even know what they are. This is an epidemic among women in many cultures. They are trained at a young age that putting others' needs before their own is the most attractive version of a mother/woman. Because of this imprinting, many women are afraid to even feel what they truly desire and certainly are afraid to express it if they do know. They fear isolation, rejection, and ultimately not being loved. In heteronormative, patriarchal cultures, a similar sentiment is true for those who do not identify as anything other than straight men. A tricky challenge is, when we do not communicate our needs clearly, we may feel like others are not respecting us or we may find ourselves yielding to their needs and then expecting them to do the same for us. We can put pressure on our loved ones to intuit what it is we want and that is an impossible expectation doomed to fail. It is a lose-lose situation fraught with frustration and resentment when we do not express what we truly desire.

Using our words to express what we need is a potent form of empowerment and the only way to have healthy relationships. There are two steps in practicing clear communication: getting clear about what we want and expressing our desires to others. It may require therapy or other supportive containers to peel back beliefs and protective layers to learn what it is we desire. This process can take time and require patience. The second step may also benefit from encouraging guidance as many fears can surface at the thought of sharing our newly discovered desires. This lifestyle tip is a practice for beginning to sense what we want.

LIFESTYLE TIP

Honoring Clear Yeses & No's

So often we feel a clear yes or a clear no about a choice that is presented to us. Even though we undoubtedly sense this, we frequently still go ahead with something that is a no and we avoid doing things that are a yes. It is incredible how many things we do each day that fit this description. I invite you to play with honoring your clear yeses and no's. Start by slowing down enough to tune into yourself before plowing ahead on autopilot. Do you actually want that cup of coffee? Do you want to eat right now? Do you want to give a hug right now? Do you want to receive feedback right now? So many of our daily actions are habituated. We do not even consider the possibility that we might not want something at that moment. You can follow up some of these inquiries with, for example, if I do not want coffee, what do I want? Also, pay attention to the full-body feeling of excitement when something is a clear yes. Whenever that happens, this is a clear indicator to go ahead even if it is something unknown or scary.

BOUNDARY SETTING

All the clients I have worked with have stagnant energy in their solar plexus, the energy center just above the navel. Anytime we feel a violation of our will or are overpowered by an authority figure, our solar plexus is affected. People of color, women, LGBTQIA+, immigrants, neurodiverse, and others that are born into the predominantly racist, heterosexist, xenophobic, patriarchal construct that pervades many cultures of our world experience countless transgressions of their will. It seems throughout history, there has consistently been the exertion of one group's will over another's. Additionally, people's personal experiences often contain numerous violations of their will. Sometimes these violations are overt, while other times they are subtly manipulative. Learning how to set clear boundaries for ourselves through awareness and healing of our specific set of transgressions is a life-changing practice.

In some cases, we are unaware of the impact that dominance being exerted upon us has. For example, as children, our caretakers did the best they knew how to care for us. Oftentimes, the way many caretakers approached parenting left us feeling unheard, with our power squashed down. Guilt and shame are frequently used as leverage to get a child to not behave a certain way again. This compounds the disempowerment. After multiple interactions like this over several years, we become programmed to fear that love will be withdrawn from us if we express our will. We learn to make ourselves small and when we do assert ourselves it is from a place of rebellious reaction rather than empowered action. Our solar plexus is home to our warrior. Having access to our willpower allows us to set clear boundaries. On the contrary, when our solar plexus has stagnant energy, we may find it difficult to be resourceful when it comes to setting boundaries. When it is really blocked, we may feel nauseous at the mere thought of setting a clear boundary.

One way to fan the flames of our willpower is to surround ourselves with people who are on a similar path of growth. These people will understand your process, and they will support and celebrate you. If we continue to expose ourselves to toxic or non-supportive relationships, we reinforce the self-limiting stories we tell ourselves. Sometimes we may not be aware that a relationship is toxic. We may need a trusted, objective perspective to help us see this clearly. Either way, if a relationship feeds off a power dynamic that keeps us small, strong boundaries need to be set or the relationship shed. It is crucial to recognize which relationships these are and to form clear boundaries about how you will or will not engage. If there is unwillingness from the other person to accept these boundaries, it is important to consider lovingly letting them go. This can be a tender topic as we may have self-judgment about what it means to withdraw from a relationship with certain people. It can be scary because you may fear that these are the only people who will love you. This is not true and will never be true. We all deserve to be in the company of people who recognize and celebrate our brilliance and our boundaries.

LIFESTYLE TIP

Your Inner Circle

- Who are the people you currently spend the most time interacting with?

- Are they supportive of your growth?

- Are they on a similar path of growth in their own lives?

- Are they good listeners?

- Do you feel acknowledged and appreciated by them?

- Do you feel like you can share your failures without judgment?

- Can you celebrate your successes with them?

These are some guiding questions that ideally you answered yes to about your inner circle. It makes all the difference to surround ourselves with people who can celebrate, support, and understand us. If you find that some (or all) of the people are no's to these questions, consider choosing a relationship with them that has clear boundaries including things such as not receiving their opinions, not sharing your dreams, and perhaps not sharing your victories and failures. We do not want to welcome people into our lives who criticize us rather than offer respectful feedback. Find new friends and mentors that mirror the ideals you want to live by. Choose wisely.

...

There are an infinite number of practices we can choose from to implement into our lives to gain new awareness, integrate, heal, and grow. The key is to do them with consistency and commitment. For the duration of our lives, we are going to want to update our practices to best match the dreams we are manifesting and the new challenges that are arising. At the conclusion of this book, there is a list of suggested modalities and books to get you started with finding support in each area of the *Wheel of Whole Body Healing*. Different times will require different resources to heal and grow. Seek out the support needed to aid each new threshold.

NINE

LIVING OUR LIFE'S PURPOSE

*Progress can be made if you are ready to take the
great leap and risk it all for the sake of love.*

RICHARD RUDD
Gene Keys

W hat is our life's purpose anyway? This phrase gets tossed
around a lot, but what does it really mean? Our life's purpose is to bring forth our greatest gifts. It is not necessarily defined
by the job we choose, though ideally, all our life circumstances are
ultimately in accordance with our purpose. It is rooted in our
heart. Its foundation is love. It is the truest form of our creative
expression. It is creating value for others. It is the essence of our
soul manifest on earth. It is discovering our desires and allowing
our life to be led by them. It is life-supporting. It is expansive. It
brings us great joy.

Malidoma Patrice Somé eloquently spoke about purpose in his
book, *The Healing Wisdom of Africa: Finding Life Purpose through
Nature, Ritual, and Community*[1]. He said, "There are two things
people crave: the full realization of their innate gifts, and to have
these gifts approved, acknowledged, and confirmed."[2] He goes on

to share the perspective of his people, the Dagara of West Africa, by saying purpose is something given before birth. All in that community know what gifts an incoming soul is bringing by the time they are born and how these gifts will serve the health of the community. Our purpose is with us all along. Our task is to remember what it is since many modern-day cultures no longer have a connection with community and Spirit to guide us and remind us of our purpose as children.

Despite the lack of community support in honoring our gifts, there are those of us who are willing to "risk it all for the sake of love" because we have a deep knowing that we belong to something greater. We will settle for nothing less than awakening this ecstatic state of being. We are anchoring a frequency of light in a world full of chaos as visionary leaders creating examples of new ways of living. It is an evolutionary spiral that is infused with the wisdom of the past and reinvented to meet the needs of our current times. As we connect more and more with the love that we are, we are better able to know and fulfill our life's purpose.

HOW FEAR SABOTAGES LIVING OUR PURPOSE

When we distill it down, physical and emotional imbalances reflect places within us still harboring fear. That is not to say the choices we make cause illnesses, syndromes, conditions, etc., though sometimes this is true. I am referring to how we choose to relate to our bodies and experience of life.

Our natural state of being is love. Many things happen to us throughout our lives that interrupt the frequency of love and shift it to fear. Some happen directly through personal life experience, and some happen indirectly via paths such as our lineage lines.

Oftentimes, we are unconscious that fear is the ruling voice of our agony. We may be aware of a particular physical or emotional state that does not feel good; however, we may not yet be ready to let go of the fear. Why? Safety is the answer. We often choose what is familiar to us even if we know it is not moving us toward our greatest potential. By doing this, we protect ourselves from the "dangerous" possibility of the unknown. We feel safe in our unconsciousness. We choose security, causing unsupportive patterns to loop and reinforce our disempowered status, rather than take a leap into love. I find the essence of this quote by Richard Rudd to be spot on,

> In the West, we no longer fear our survival because we have created a society that supports everyone at the collective level... Because of this, our fear has shifted to a fear of purposelessness. Now instead of being afraid to die, people are afraid to live... Most people do not even want to think about whether they are fulfilling their true purpose or not because to do so is to look right into their deepest fears.[3]

We have many wounds, or places lacking love, that exist in our physical bodies and our emotional bodies. It does not have to be grueling and intense to address these wounds. They do not need to be tackled one by one throughout our lives to feel good. On the contrary, as we acknowledge the truth that our fears are the root cause of our suffering, our consciousness changes. It can change very quickly. We then begin to see exponential results in our bodies and our lives. This type of healing is not simply about correcting physical pain. It is taking a quantum leap. It affects all areas of our lives. When we acknowledge our current circumstances are "serving" the part of us that is terrified of the unknown, we can make different choices, and monumental change follows.

Taking responsibility can be a tough pill to swallow. It is not a path for the faint-hearted. Truth be told, historically few have taken this path of empowerment. But we live in a different time now. We are in a critical hour with climate crisis upon us, species of plants and animals becoming endangered/extinct daily, growing dead zones in the oceans, global pandemics occurring, outmoded systems breaking down, etc. The way we have been doing things is destroying the planet, and us along with it. We need a collective quantum leap to begin re-establishing the equilibrium.

There are enough of us who are excited to rise up and heal by remembering and living the truth of who we are. We are willing to plunge into the shadows and see what resides there. We are dedicated to looking defeat in the eye and choosing to not settle for anything less than the most fully expressed version of ourselves. We believe in the greater good of humanity.

This movement anchors a higher vibration in the collective consciousness of the global human population. When we add in the children being born with a different framework that ushers in a new consciousness, it weighs the scales towards a tipping point. Every day, we are inspiring one another to grow and expand. We are finding forgiveness for ourselves and others. We see failure as opportunities, rather than reasons to be punished. We have courage to express our creative genius and share our gifts with others. We know that we matter; and no matter how grand or small our gestures are, they matter. The more we embody the understanding that everything is interconnected, and everyone impacts everything, the more we find fuel to bear the discomfort of meeting our fears. Unless we are in a moment of physical harm, the stories our fear tells us are cries for help from neglected parts of ourselves yearning for attention. When we approach fear with curiosity, we can make empowered choices and stop looking outside ourselves to be fixed or healed. As we meet ourselves with love, we soften into our divine essence, accepting the perfection of who we are. In the still point, where judgment does not exist, we are nothing more and nothing less than love.

THE IMPORTANCE OF LIVING OUR LIFE'S PURPOSE

Committing to love is at the core of living our life's purpose. It evolves our consciousness, as well as that of humanity. Embodying love restores us to wholeness, vitality, and joy. What this looks like is different for every one of us. Some qualities include treating ourselves and one another with kindness, reverence, and appreciation. It is the small victories of choosing love that allow greater access to joy and freedom in our daily lives.

We all want to experience freedom in the deepest sense of the word, freedom from feeling isolated, unworthy, unloveable... The list goes on and on. To experience freedom, we need to embrace our life's purpose and live it.

We *all* have come here with a purpose that serves humanity. Each one of us has unique gifts that are a necessary contribution to this beautiful co-creation of life on Earth. We are all special and our soul's wisdom is needed. We can choose to spend our whole lives tricking ourselves into believing lies based on the fear that we are insignificant and unworthy. But why? And at what cost?

SERVICE AND CONTRIBUTION = JOY

If our primary purpose is to evolve as a species, and by this, I mean spiritually as well as physically, we must begin to acknowledge the unique brilliance that resides within each human. We must identify our gifts and be willing to share them as our service and contribution to humanity. It is here that we will find our greatest joy. Joy does not come from outside ourselves. It does not come from a relationship, money, or a nice house to live in. It comes from a deep understanding that we are all connected, there is no separation, and therefore we are intimately connected to all that exists.

Ask yourself these questions,

- When are the times you have experienced the greatest joy in your life thus far?

- What specifically were you doing?

- Were you of service to another life?

- Were you in deep communion with Spirit through nature, meditation, or giving birth?

The answers to these questions are clues as to what we need to do *more* of in our lives. They are the activities we need to prioritize even if it seems to not fit into our schedules or make logical sense. It is not simply the doing of the activities, but rather the quality of presence we bring. If we listen to our hearts and follow the actions that make us feel most alive, we will inevitably be living a fuller expression of our life's purpose. In the choice to follow our truest desires, we are of service. Sometimes it may not be obvious that we are being of service. However, we contribute to humanity regardless of what we are doing when we embody the presence of being. When we choose love as our guiding light, we are making the most magnificent contribution of all.

EXERCISE

Finding Joy & Purpose

There are many clues to knowing if we are on the right path to discovering and expressing our life's purpose. Ask yourself these questions as you go through your day.

- How do I feel when I'm doing certain activities or with certain people?

- Does it bring me joy? Or discomfort, frustration, or depression?

- Does it feel easy? Or do I feel like I am pushing every step along the way?

- Do I feel inspired and hungry for more?

- Am I being helpful to another without needing anything in return?

A helpful clue is, do you feel a sense of ease and flow? If you are laboring over something or doing a project that feels tiresome and efforted your intentions likely need re-evaluating. Begin to recognize the uplifting activities versus the ones that feel draining.

...

Discovering our life's purpose need not be an overwhelming event or one we put pressure on ourselves to uncover. On the contrary, I invite it to be an easeful inquiry inspired by that which touches your heart and rocks your soul. There are no rules here. There is no correct way for our life's purpose to look or be. If thoughts like this arise, it may be someone else's voice we have adopted as our own placing a measure on our value by the external "successes" of our lives. It may also be some of our wounded selves comparing us to other people and what brings them apparent joy. We are the only ones who can truly know what brings us pleasure, joy, happiness, and ecstasy. If we approach our ever-unfolding life's purpose with levity, play, curiosity, and non-judgment, we can spontaneously discover new things that inspire us. Then, with our inspiration, we can make brilliant creations that touch the hearts of others.

TEN

REMEMBERING OUR MAGNIFICENCE

Our deepest fear is not that we are inadequate.
Our deepest fear is that we are powerful beyond measure.
It is our light, not our darkness that most frightens us.
We ask ourselves, Who am I to be brilliant,
gorgeous, talented, fabulous?
Actually, who are you not to be?
You are a child of God.
Your playing small
doesn't serve the world.

MARIANNE WILLIAMSON
A Return to Love

EVOLVING OUR PERCEPTION OF SELF

Pain is part of the human experience. It is not possible to eliminate all pain. However, we do not have to suffer. We can change our relationship to suffering. Changing our relationship to suffering and redefining our relationship to healing happen simultaneously. As we begin to understand that healing is a transformational journey and not equivalent to a condition ceasing to exist or be cured, our relationship to suffering radically shifts. We come to realize that we can even experience healing in our final breaths. We grasp that healing does not mean a return to how our body was before, but a progressive acquiring of greater awareness and integration.

The *Wheel of Whole Body Healing*, at its heart, is a framework for an experiential exploration of the multi-layered human experience. Our health and vitality are influenced by many factors, including, but not limited to, the physical. The unseen influences of energy and emotions have a profound impact on the state of our health. Even though they are unseen, it does not mean they are inaccessible. When these factors are not taken into consideration while devising a healing plan, we are leaving out a crucial part of what causes imbalance.

As we open to the possibility that our physical symptoms are an extension of imbalances in our energy fields, we begin to have access to healing at a fundamental level. We then relate to ourselves as a version much closer to the truth; we are energetic beings currently residing in a house of bones, tissues, fluids, and organs. Exploring the various aspects of ourselves that comprise the *Wheel* offers hope through an embodied understanding of what is happening within us. Though we will need support from different professionals along the way, when we cultivate a deeper listening to our bodies and our needs, we become the captains at the helm of our glorious ships.

LISTENING TO OUR BODIES TALK

The *Wheel of Whole Body Healing* invites us to cultivate refinement of our listening skills through our senses to decipher the incredible wisdom our bodies hold. There are no right or wrong ways to do this. The exercises contained in this book are suggestions for getting started. Though it may be subtle at times, so subtle we can easily dismiss the beckoning whispers, the expression of our bodies is always present. As we learn to understand our body's unique language, it can change everything. We are no longer in the dark. Instead, we reside in a place of possibility. We learn how to skillfully hold the dualities of the healing process. For example, we may simultaneously experience physical pain *and* joy. We become empowered to support this journey of life as one of healing through growth infused with love.

The exercises in this book are self-care practices that can serve us in each stage of our evolution. As we explore applying the *Wheel*, we can begin to have a more comprehensive understanding of the symptoms we are experiencing. From this place of foundational awareness, we can make empowered choices about our healthcare support teams and take full charge of our healing.

THE IMPACT OF THE WHEEL ON COMMUNITY HEALTHCARE

When "I" is replaced with "We" even "Illness" becomes "Wellness."
MALCOLM X

The *Wheel of Whole Body Healing* serves as a template for wellness. As we become more intimate and consciously engaged with the various aspects of the *Wheel*, we become increasingly attuned with how to tend to ourselves. This is an ever-unfolding process that will endure throughout our lifetimes. It is a practice that expands as we gain a deeper understanding of our complexities. As more people redefine their relationship to healing through increased awareness of themselves, the grassroots healthcare revolution gains significant momentum.

As our perspective shifts, we engage with our health and wellness providers from a place of confidence, leadership, and co-creatorship. This flips the hierarchical power dynamic of practitioner-patient on its head. No longer are we seeking all the answers from doctors/practitioners. Instead, we are listening within and trusting our bodies and intuitions. We then bring this information to practitioners that best fit what we need. We interview them for the job of joining our healthcare team. We become fierce advocates for our wellness.

Something unique about the *Wheel of Whole Body Healing* is that it can be applied by individuals, *and* it can be implemented by community clinics, doctor's offices, and even larger healthcare systems. It is scalable. It works from the inside out (embodied individuals in an empowered collaboration with their healthcare practitioners) *and* the outside in (receptive healthcare professionals implementing the *Wheel* framework for patient care).

Additionally, the *Wheel of Whole Body Healing* is a guide for every human. It is not specific to those experiencing chronic health symptoms. Every one of us can continue to develop increased awareness and connection with our bodies, emotional tendencies, and energetic nature within the context of being spiritual beings.

During this time of collective transition related to health and healing, how do we hold the duality of new awareness gained and doctors, health insurance, etc. not being onboard with our requests? It requires creativity, persistence, and innovation. Working with the exercises in this book will help to develop trust and confidence that will allow us to weather the storm of doubt, criticism, and disbelief that may come from professionals that are unwilling to expand their points of view. In the meantime, do not compromise your values. Find practitioners who will listen and happily be part of your team. Seek community that is on a similar path of rediscovery with their relationship to healing. Many people already exist, some newly seeing the gaps in the conventional medicine paradigm and others who have long been on the journey of remembering our innate capacity to heal. This movement is here, and it is rapidly growing. We are not alone. As we drop into a deeper state of listening to ourselves and to one another, the visibility of those on this path will become apparent.

The purpose of this book is not to critique the conventional medicine paradigm. It is to provide an option for the ways this paradigm is failing. Although there are many strengths to the conventional medical model, there are great flaws as well. One of those is attempting to treat certain chronic illnesses and symptoms that the system and its practitioners are ill-equipped to handle. It is a lose-lose situation for all. This has left many people feeling a sense of isolation and hopelessness.

We are looking in the wrong place for answers. The answers lie within us. A host of lifestyle habits and beliefs are making us a nation of illness. This can only be remedied by a thorough reorientation. When we choose to take this journey of intimacy and exploration with ourselves, we uplift our communities along with us.

EXERCISE

Spreading Kindness

There are many approaches to the Loving-Kindness meditation born of the Buddhist tradition. It is a blessing that offers yourself kindness that you then extend out to others. This version is inspired by the practice in Radhule Weininger's book, *Heartwork*.[1] Feel free to modify it in any way that feels most resonant to you.

1. Take the time to ground yourself into your breath and body.

2. When you are ready, shift your attention to your heart. You may want to place your hand on your heart center. Sometimes I place my other hand over my belly button (the lower Dantian energy center).

3. Connect with the felt sense of love and kindness by stating intentions such as:

   - May my heart be full of love and kindness.
   - May my heart and mind be free from sticky thoughts and feelings.
   - May I accept my life with all its challenges and opportunities.
   - May I hold myself with gentleness and friendship.
   - May I experience peace and ease in my body.
   - May I find the support I need.
   - May we forgive ourselves and one another.

- May we have the courage to express our desires.
- May all beings be free from suffering.
- May we experience freedom and exaltation.

WE CHOOSE LOVE

The *Wheel of Whole Body Healing* is one of many frameworks that encourages us to become empowered in our healthcare journeys and in our lives. It does not matter *how* we come to better understand the true nature of healing, just that we do. As we embrace the paradox of simultaneously holding hope and hopelessness in our hearts without trying to change or fix it, a transformation occurs. When we do not make hopelessness wrong or hope right, we unburden ourselves from the weight of measuring our success as related to the linear continuum of no hope to hope. We are experiencing everything, always. As we soften into the truth of this the harshness of judgment melts away and an opening is created making way for love.

It is crucial for us, our communities, and the health of the planet to expand our perspective on what contributes to illness, what it means to heal, and how we approach healing. Although we are in an immense state of imbalance as a global community, there are options, that when implemented into our lives will radically improve our quality of life and everyone surrounding us. Whether we are aware of it or not, we sense, perceive, and feel everything; we are energetic beings. Every choice made with love, moving toward love, and opening to love is an act of revival for all. My hope is that something in this book sparked a fire within that will continuously increase in magnitude and be a steady burn throughout your life as you unfold ever more graciously into love.

Let us bring forth our greatest gifts brilliant ones

and find the courage to dive deeper into love.

Let us surround ourselves with others willing to hold us

and support us on our journeys out of fear.

Let our sincere voices reverberate our truths

even when others do not seem to understand.

Let us discover the truth of who we are within our hearts

as we hold our heads high.

Let our songs grace our ears with their unique beauty

that only our souls can create.

Let us be bold and courageous

as

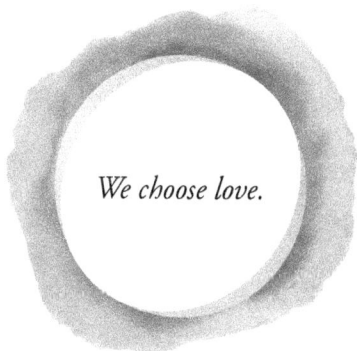

We choose love.

ACKNOWLEDGMENTS

Susan Kerr, thank you for always believing in me and encouraging me to share my work with the world. I can hear your glorious laughter celebrating the completion of this book. May your love shine down from the stars and bless all who are guided to read this book.

Azeza and Luciana, thank you for inspiring me to stick to the task of ever-expanding my capacity to give and receive love. May you always see the goodness in this world and recognize it reflecting back to you your inextinguishable light.

Emily Cashwell, words cannot convey my depth of appreciation for you. It is through your eyes I repeatedly found my way back to the essence of this book's message. You witnessed and uplifted me every step along the way. Thank you for being my rock, upholder of integrity, and always asking the correct questions. Your friendship means the world to me. May every person be so blessed to have someone as devoted to authentic expression in their life as you.

Vanessa Owen, thank you for mirroring how to be a more skillful listener. Your brilliance and loving heart contributed to bringing this book into greater alignment. I am deeply grateful for your willingness to come blazing in during the final hour.

Linsey Dodaro, thank you for gracing this project with your creative genius and impeccable eye. What a gift to have this project imbued with your energy.

Emilie Bers, thank you for a magical and empowering photo shoot. Something shifted in me that day that touched my heart and forever changed me.

Marla Mattenson, thank you for being a torchbearer on the path of integrity and reflecting my light to me. You are a wise teacher and guide that I am honored to walk alongside and bear witness to.

Gina Belton, thank you for introducing me to wisdom teachers that have opened my heart and expanded my perspective. Your guidance has increased my capacity for kindness, reciprocity, and generosity.

Lily Robertson, our time together has transformed me. You are a great gift in my life. Thank you for being part of my team.

Devi and Carlos, thank you for believing in this project and supporting it with your kind words.

This book is the physical manifestation of a labor of love. Along the way, there have been many who have inspired me to keep going and reminded me of the importance of this message. To all these people, including former clients who entrusted me with being their guide, I appreciate you.

NOTES

FOREWORD

1. C. Buttorff, T. Ruder, and M. Bauman, "Multiple Chronic Conditions in the United States," (Santa Monica, CA: Rand Corp, 2017), https://www.rand.org/content/dam/rand/pubs/tools/TL200/TL221/RAND_TL221.pdf.

2. Johns Hopkins School of Public Health and Robert Wood Johnson Foundation, "Chronic Conditions: Making the Case for Ongoing Care." PowerPoint Presentation, February 2010, https://smhs.gwu.edu/sites/default/files/ChronicCareChartbook.pdf.

3. Centers for Disease Control (CDC), *About the Center* (Atlanta, GA: CDC, 2023), https://www.cdc.gov/chronicdisease/center/index.htm.

4. Centers for Disease Control (CDC), *Health and Economic Costs of Chronic Diseases* (Atlanta, GA: CDC, 2022), https://www.cdc.gov/chronicdisease/about/costs/index.htm.

CHAPTER TWO

1. To learn more about Dr. Peter Levine and his body of work, *Somatic Experiencing*, visit www.traumahealing.org.

2. Peter A. Levine, *Waking the Tiger: Healing Trauma* (Berkley, CA: North Atlantic Books, 1997).

3. Levine, *Waking the Tiger*, 19.

4. Richard C. Schwartz, *No Bad Parts: Healing Trauma and Restoring Wholeness with the Internal Family Systems Model* (Boulder, CO: Sounds True, 2021).

5. Bradley Nelson, *Emotion Code: How to Release Your Trapped Emotions for Abundant Health, Love, and Happiness* (New York: St. Martin's Essentials, 2019).

6. Brené Brown, *Atlas of the Heart: Mapping Meaningful Connection and the Language of the Human Experience* (New York: Random House, 2021).

7. To learn more about Dr. Donny Epstein's revolutionary body of work *Network Spinal Analysis* visit www.epienergetics.com or visit a Network Chiropractor near you.

CHAPTER THREE

1. Suzy Amis Cameron, *The OMD Plan: Swap One Meal a Day to Save Your Health and Save the Planet* (New York: Atria, 2019).

2. Only Organic, "How to Make Organic Food Accessible and Affordable for Everyone," Organic News, November 5, 2020, https://www.onlyorganic.org/how-to-make-organic-accessible-and-affordable-for-everyone/.

3. John Fagan et al. "Organic Diet Intervention Significantly Reduces Urinary Glyphosate Levels in U.S. Children and Adults." *Environmental Research* 189, (2020): 1-7. https://doi.org/10.1016/j.envres.2020.109898.

4. Only Organic, "How to Make Organic Food Accessible and Affordable for Everyone."

5. Kristen D'Amato, *FOOD for the light body: Simple plant-based & gluten-free recipes for the body & soul* (Asheville, NC: 2017).

CHAPTER FOUR

1. To find out more about Charlie Goldsmith visit www.charliegoldsmith.com.

2. Clinton Ober et al., Earthing: The Most Important Health Discovery Ever! (Basic HealthPublications, 2014).

CHAPTER FIVE

1. Shamini Jain, *Healing Ourselves: Biofield Science and the Future of Health* (Boulder, CO: Sounds True, 2021).

2. Jain, *Healing Ourselves*, 18.

3. Beverly Rubik et al. "Biofield Science and Healing: History, Terminology, and Concepts." *Global Advances in Health and Medicine* 4, 1_suppl, (2015): 6, https://www.doi.org/10.7453/gahmj.2015.038.suppl.

4. Drunvalo Melchizedek, *Living in the Heart* (Light Technology Publishing, 2003).

5. Rollin McCraty, "The Energetic Heart: Bioelectromagnetic Communication Within and Between People," in *Clinical Applications of Bioelectromagnetic Medicine*, ed. P. J. Rosch and M. S. Markov (New York: Marcel Dekker, 2004), 541-562.

6. Barrie Sands. "Overview of the Heart's Intelligence: A Dynamic Perspective into the World of Energetic Wellness." *Journal of the American Holistic Veterinary Medical Association* 68, (Fall 2022), 22-30, https://www.doi.org/10.56641/LDSI6326.

7. Sands, "Overview of the Heart's Intelligence," 23.

8. For more information about the HeartMath Institute visit www.hearthmath.org.

9. To see an image of the toroidal field around the heart visit www.heartmath.org/research/science-of-the-heart/energetic-communication/ or type "toroidal field around the heart images" in Google search.

CHAPTER SIX

1. Levine, *Waking the Tiger*, 39.

2. Stanislav Zhdanov, "Unity Breath Meditation by Drunvalo Melchizedek," YouTube, January 24, 2014, https://www.youtube.com/watch?v=NFfMuOr95AA.

CHAPTER SEVEN

1. Tami Lynn Kent, *Wild Feminine: Finding Power, Spirit, and Joy in the Female Body* (New York: Atria, 2011).

2. To learn more about Marla Mattenson's work visit her website at www.marlamattenson.com.

3. Kasia Urbaniak, *Unbound: A Woman's Guide to Her Power* (New York: Tarcher Perigree, 2021).

4. Mantak Chia and Maneewan Chia, *Healing Love through the Tao: Cultivating Female Sexual Energy* (Rochester, VT: Destiny Books, 2005).

5. Mantak Chia and Michael Winn, *Taoist Secrets of Love: Cultivating Male Sexual Energy* (Aurora Press, 1984).

CHAPTER NINE

1. Malidoma Patrice Somé, *The Healing Wisdom of Africa: Finding Life Purpose through Nature, Ritual, and Community* (New York: Tarcher Putman, 1998).

2. Somé, *The Healing Wisdom of Africa*, 27.

3. Richard Rudd, *Gene Keys: Embracing your Higher Purpose* (London: Watkins, 2013), 220.

CHAPTER TEN

1. Radhule Weininger, *Heartwork: The Path of Self-Compassion* (Boulder, CO: Shambala, 2017), 67.

HEALING MODALITIES & RESOURCES

Here is a list including some of the *many* incredible resources available. Some of the modalities are applicable to multiple aspects of the *Wheel of Whole Body Healing*.

UNEXPRESSED EMOTIONAL ENERGY

Books & Resources:
The Body Keeps the Score by Bessel van der Kolk
Waking the Tiger by Peter Levine
The Wild Edge of Sorrow by Francis Weller
No Bad Parts by Richard Schwartz
Atlas of the Heart by Brené Brown
Attached. by Amir Levine & Rachel Heller

Modalities:
Network Chiropractic (Network Spinal Analysis)
EMDR (eye-movement desensitization reprocessing)
Internal Family Systems Therapy
Somatic Experiencing
Psychotherapy
Mindfulness Meditation
Clinical hypnosis
Box breathing
Grief Rituals
Expressive Journaling
Martial Arts

DIET & NUTRITION

Books & Resources:
Food for the Light Body by Kristen D'Amato
Liver Rescue by Anthony William
Cleanse to Heal by Anthony William
OMD by Suzy Cameron
The Way of Miracles by Mark Mincolla, Ph.D. (book and film)
Cowspiracy: The Sustainability Secret – film
What the Health – documentary film
Eating Our Way to Extinction – documentary film
Forks Over Knives – documentary film
High quality supplements – www.vimergy.com
Anthony Williams – www.medicalmedium.com

Modalities:
Holistic Nutrition Coach
Ayurvedic Nutritionist

PHYSICAL AILMENTS & IMBALANCES

Books & Resources:
No Bad Parts by Richard Schwartz
Sensing, Feeling, and Action by Bonnie Bainbridge Cohen
Earthing by Ober, Zucker, and Sinatra
Breath by James Nestor
Body-Mind Centering - www.bodymindcentering.com

Modalities:
Medical Intuitive
Integrative Medicine

Body-Mind Centering
Acupuncture
Clinical hypnosis/Self-Hypnosis
Yoga, Tai Chi, Qi Gong
Authentic Movement
4-7-8 breathing technique

THE ENERGY FIELD

Books & Resources:
Hands of Light by Barbara Ann Brennan
Healing Ourselves: Biofield Science and the Future of Health by
    Shamini Jain
The Mastery Trilogy by Paul Selig
The Seven Spiritual Laws of Success by Deepak Chopra
Unity Breath Meditation by Drunvalo Melchizedek
The HeartMath Institute - www.heartmath.com

Modalities:
Visionary Craniosacral Work
Qigong Healing/ Medical Qigong
Vipassana Meditation
Reiki
Healing Touch Therapy
Quantum-Touch
Sound Healing

HEALING OUR ANCESTRAL LINEAGES

Books & Resources:
It Didn't Start with You by Mark Wolynn
Mother Hunger by Kelly McDaniel
Connecting to Our Ancestral Past by Francesca Mason Boring
Emotional Inheritance by Galit Atlas
Boys Will Be Human by Justin Baldoni (for parents)
Codependent No More by Melody Beattie
Connect with Your Ancestors by Patricia Kathleen Robertson
Ancestral Healing for Your Spiritual and Genetic Families by Jeanne Ruland & Shantidevi
Healing Ancestral Trauma by Stephen Farmer
Root & Ritual by Becca Piastrelli

Modalities:
Hand-in-Hand Parenting (for parents)
Psychic Mediumship
Shamanic Journeying
Family Constellation
Psychic Healing

EMBODYING OUR SEXUAL POWER

Books & Resources:
Women's Anatomy of Arousal by Sheri Winston
Wild Feminine by Tami Lynn Kent
Mating in Captivity: Unlocking Erotic Intelligence by Esther Perel
Womb Awakening by Azra Bertrand and Seren Bertrand
Come As You Are by Emily Nagaski

Conscious Cock by Kristopher Lovestone
Unbound by Kasia Urbaniak
Healing Love through the Tao: Cultivating Female Sexual Energy by Mantak Chia & Maneewan Chia
Taoist Secrets of Love: Cultivating Male Sexual Energy by Mantak Chia
Getting the Love You Want by Harville Hendrix

Modalities:
Holistic Pelvic Health Care
Sex Coaching
Intimacy/Relationship Coaching
Tantric Dance
Mercier Therapy
Bellydance
Maya Abdominal Massage
Rites of Passage Experiences

EMPOWERMENT TOOLS & STRATEGIES

Books & Resources:
The Embodied Mind by Thomas Verny
Breaking the Habit of Being Yourself by Joe Dispenza
Ask and It Is Given by Esther and Jerry Hicks

LIVING OUR LIFE'S PURPOSE

Books & Resources:
The Healing Wisdom of Africa: Finding Life Purpose through Nature, Ritual, and Community by Malidoma Patrice Somé

Gene Keys by Richard Rudd

Standing at the Edge: Finding Where Freedom and Courage Meet by Joan Halifax

Human Design: Discover the Person You Were Born to Be by Chetan Parkyn

Modalities:
Human design sessions
Life Coaching

REMEMBERING OUR MAGNIFICENCE

Books & Resources:
The Gift - Poetry of Hafiz – translated by Daniel Ladinsky
The Four Agreements by Don Miguel Ruiz
Heartwork by Radhule Weininger
A Radical Awakening by Dr. Shefali
The Untethered Soul by Michael Singer

Modalities:
Loving kindness meditation

EXERCISES & LIFESTYLE TIPS

Listening Within – Sensing Subtle Energy – Ch. 1
Dialoguing With Your Inner Selves – Ch. 2
Tuning In with Your Emotions - Ch. 2
List of Emotional States – Ch. 2
What Am I Making This Mean? – Ch. 2
One Meal a Day – Ch. 3
Spring Recipe – Tuscan Tempeh – Ch. 3
Summer Recipe – Romaine Leaf Tacos with Sundried Tomatoes, Lacinato Kale, & Blue Potatoes – Ch. 3
Autumn Recipe – Purple Top Turnip Thai Coconut Curry – Ch. 3
Winter Recipe – Portuguese Kale Soup – Ch. 3
Listening to Your Pain – Ch. 4
Grounding Emotional Energy – Ch. 4
Breathing Love into Your Pain – Ch. 4
Sensing Your Heart's Toroidal Field – Ch. 5
Activating Your Energy Field – Ch. 5
Releasing Ritual – Ch. 5
Support from Your Ancestors – Ch. 6
Connecting With Your Higher Self & Spirit Guides – Ch. 6
Make a New Choice – Ch. 6
Energetic Womb Cleansing – Ch. 7
Just Ask – Ch. 7
Non-Gender Specific Self-Pleasure Practice – Ch. 7
Exploring Your Wild Side – Ch. 7
Imagining the Life You Desire – Ch.8

ABOUT THE AUTHOR

Kristen D'Amato believes every person has valuable gifts and talents that contribute to the well-being of the global community. Upliftment is at the heart of all the work she shares.

Over a decade ago, Kristen created the *Wheel of Whole Body Healing*, a health and wellness model that places the power of wellness back into the hands, hearts, and minds of the individual so they can become confident co-creators in their healing journey. This evolving model has deeply impacted the lives of those who have integrated the philosophy of the *Wheel* into their lives. Kristen is the founder and CEO of *Come to Life*, a business dedicated to inspiring change in healthcare through educating providers and patients about the *Wheel of Whole Body Healing*.

Kristen earned a bachelor's degree in music theory and composition, and painting. She earned her master's degree in mind-body medicine with a certificate in contemplative end-of-life care. Her doctoral research, in the field of mind-body medicine, explores themes of belonging, grief, and how a perceived lack of belonging contributes to chronic conditions.

In addition to her work with *Come to Life*, Kristen has guided women for several years through facilitating grief rituals and practices that help them feel more at home in their bodies. She completed a 500-hour certification in sex and relationship coaching and is a trained energy medicine practitioner.

Her first book, *Food for the Light Body: Simple plant-based & gluten-free recipes for the body & soul* is a cookbook that offers a seasonal collection of fast, simple-to-make recipes inspired by cuisine around the globe. It is the culmination of one of Kristen's earlier businesses that provided nourishing, accessible meals to her local community and education about using food as medicine.

Kristen is a plant-based artist, conservationist, rebel heart, and mother of two gorgeous children. She currently resides oceanside in Los Angeles.

To learn more, visit kristendamato.com.

ABOUT COME TO LIFE

Our mission at Come to Life is to uplift, empower, and teach others to consciously co-create with their body's innate ability to heal through education, listening, acceptance, kindness, and love. Our work is grounded in transformation through embodiment. We guide others toward a sense of absolute belonging to their bodies, to their communities, to each other, and to our planet.

You can learn more about Come to Life at wecometolife.com.

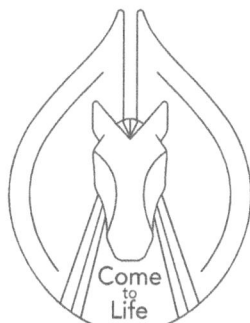

www.ingramcontent.com/pod-product-compliance
Lightning Source LLC
Chambersburg PA
CBHW022054020426
42335CB00012B/686